SOMATIC THERAPY SOLUTION

STRESS-FREE TOOLS AND EXERCISES TO MANAGE TRAUMA, PTSD, AND ANXIETY; SOOTHE CHRONIC PAIN; AND STRENGTHEN THE MIND-BODY CONNECTION FOR AN EMPOWERED LIFE

MADELINE MILLS

CONTENTS

a FREE gift

just for you

Thank you for choosing Somatic Therapy Solution. As a way of supporting your journey from the very first page, I'm thrilled to offer you an exclusive bonus: the *Panic Attack Survival Guide*—absolutely free. This guide is packed with practical, grounding tools to help you manage intense moments with ease and confidence.

To access your free guide, just scan the QR code below and enjoy instant support on your healing journey. It's my way of saying thank you for investing in your well-being and trusting me as a guide along the way.

**For your FREE
Panic Attack Survival Guide:
Scan Here**

This exclusive guide is completely FREE. Just one quick scan, and you'll have instant access to tools and strategies specifically designed to help you navigate and manage panic attacks.

It's FREE – Peace of Mind Included!

INTRODUCTION

Several years ago, I reached a pivotal moment in my life. A traumatic event left me feeling disconnected from my body, with anxiety and chronic pain constantly shadowing me. If you've ever felt estranged from yourself and weighed down by emotional or physical pain—know that you are not ever alone.

I remember struggling to sleep, waking up in the middle of the night with my mind racing, stressing about *everything*. On days of high anxiety, focusing felt impossible, which made it difficult to show up fully as the mom and wife I wanted to be. Conventional therapies provided some relief, but something was missing.

It wasn't until I discovered somatic therapy that I found the missing piece of the puzzle.

What if the key to healing isn't just in your mind—but in your body as well? This idea transformed everything for me. As I began practicing somatic therapy, my body slowly released the deep-seated tension I hadn't even realized I was holding. It felt as though an invisible weight had been lifted from my shoulders, allowing me to breathe more freely.

I wrote this book to support people who are navigating trauma, PTSD, anxiety, and chronic pain. My hope is that these pages offer you lasting relief and a sense of renewed peace. Having experienced the life-changing power of somatic therapy firsthand, I share here these transformative tools with you—a steady compass to help you find your way toward healing and wholeness.

Somatic therapy offers a way for you to heal by tuning into your body's sensations and using them as a guide for transformation. At its core is the understanding that trauma isn't just a mental or emotional experience—it's stored in the body, too. By becoming aware of the physical sensations connected to trauma, we can begin to process and release the pain held within us.

Think of your body as a library. Every experience—whether a cherished memory or a traumatic event—is stored, like a page, within your muscles, breath, and posture, waiting to be read and understood. Just as you wouldn't skip pages of an important book, somatic therapy teaches us to pay attention to each sensation and emotion.

The purpose of this book is simple: to make these powerful practices accessible to everyone. You'll find actionable steps, exercises, and a customizable 28-day healing program to help you build a stronger connection between your mind and body. My goal is to equip you with the tools you can use *every day* to foster resilience, ease, and personal empowerment.

So, why is somatic therapy so important?

Trauma, PTSD, anxiety, and chronic pain don't just affect our mind; they leave a lasting imprint on our body, altering our nervous systems and actually leading to physical symptoms. Research shows that somatic therapy effectively reduces symptoms of trauma and anxiety by addressing these imprints holistically, promoting healing on every level.

Each chapter in this book explores a specific healing area, with practical exercises you can integrate into your daily routine. Think of this book as a map through a dense forest—each chapter offers a trail to follow, tools to use, and rest points along the way.

Several key themes run throughout these pages. First, the exercises are trauma-informed, ensuring they are safe and supportive. We will explore holistic practices integrating physical, mental, and emotional healing—such as yoga, Tai Chi, and Pilates. Mindfulness techniques will help you build emotional resilience and develop a deeper awareness of your body. Finally, we'll focus on self-compassion, a vital element in the healing process.

Who is this book written for?

It's for anyone struggling with trauma, PTSD, anxiety, or chronic pain. It's for those seeking to strengthen their mind–body connection. You'll discover practical exercises, but the way you engage with them will be uniquely your style—there's no one-size-fits-all approach. Whether you're new to somatic therapy or have some prior experience, you'll find valuable insights and practical tools here.

What makes this book unique is its interactive and customizable approach. Throughout the chapters, you'll encounter journaling prompts and reflection exercises designed to actively engage you in your healing journey. Self-assessment tools will help you track your progress and make any adjustments as needed.

Let's take this journey together! Think of healing as a garden you nurture—each mindful breath, compassionate act, and moment of self-reflection is a seed planted. It's essential to honor where you are in your healing process. Just like you wouldn't push a sprouting plant to grow *faster*, somatic therapy encourages gentle, supportive growth. Go at your own pace—healing happens one step at a time. With time and care, those seeds will bloom into strength, peace, and empowerment. You already have the strength, tools, and support to heal.

This path is uniquely yours, but you don't have to walk it alone. I'll be with you, step by step, as you transform the inevitable challenges into opportunities for growth. Together, we'll uncover the tools to reconnect with your body, and build a life of balance, rooted in healing.

Healing isn't really a destination—it's a journey. Imagine you're hiking through a dense forest. Some days, the path is clear, and other times, it's hidden beneath overgrowth. Healing can feel just the same—it requires patience, presence, and trust that even when the trail seems obscured, progress is still being made—and you have everything you need to navigate it.

Let's begin.

1

FOUNDATIONS OF SOMATIC THERAPY

Have you ever felt like your body is carrying a weight you can't explain—like you're bracing for impact, even though nothing is happening? I know that feeling well. There was a time when every muscle in my body felt tense, as if I were stuck in a perpetual state of readiness, waiting for something to go wrong. Sleep was elusive, and anxiety weighed heavily on me, making it hard to be the mom and wife I wanted to be.

It wasn't until I discovered somatic therapy that I learned my body was actually holding on to trauma. This was a revelation—suddenly I understood that the tension wasn't at all random, and with that understanding came the hope of relief. What had once felt like an insoluble burden began to feel *manageable.* The aches and pains had a name, and even more importantly, there was a way forward.

This chapter lays the foundation for understanding how somatic therapy works and why it can profoundly impact your healing journey.

1.1 UNDERSTANDING SOMATIC THERAPY: PRINCIPLES AND PRACTICES

Somatic therapy is a body-centered approach that focuses on the physical sensations in your body as a pathway to emotional healing. The term "somatic" means "relating to the body." Unlike traditional "talk therapy", e.g., psychoanalysis, which primarily engages the mind, somatic therapy uses awareness, movement, and touch to help you process and release stored trauma. Our bodies store memories of traumatic events, and by becoming aware of these sensations, we can begin to heal from within.

At its core, somatic therapy *brings you back into your body*—teaching you to listen to its whispers before they become shouts.

Unresolved emotions can block your ability to flow through life with ease. Imagine your body as a river, and these emotions as fallen branches and debris blocking the current. Over time, the water becomes stagnant and cloudy. Somatic therapy helps clear these blockages, allowing the river to flow freely again—restoring clarity, movement, and vitality.

The body-centered somatic therapy approach isn't new—its roots run deep through Eastern and Western traditions. For centuries, Eastern philosophies have recognized the mind–body connection, integrating physical practices like yoga and Tai Chi to promote overall well-being. In the West, somatic therapy gained traction through the work of pioneers like Dr. Peter Levine, who developed Somatic Experiencing; and Ron Kurtz, who created the Hakomi Method. These modalities have evolved to include Sensorimotor Psychotherapy, which combines elements of traditional psychotherapy with body-focused techniques.

Somatic Experiencing focuses on helping individuals become aware of physical sensations linked to trauma. By feeling these sensations in manageable increments—a process known as titration—you can gradually release stored energy. Then there's the Hakomi Method, which uses mindfulness and gentle touch to explore unconscious beliefs that affect your body, and your emotions.

Sensorimotor Psychotherapy, on the other hand, integrates attachment theory and neuroscience to address how past physical experiences influence current behavior and emotional states.

The goals of somatic therapy are broad, yet deeply personal. One primary objective is emotional and physical healing. You can understand and release emotional pain by paying attention to bodily sensations. Another goal is to enhance body awareness, helping you become more attuned to the signals your body sends. This heightened awareness aids in building resilience and self-regulation, enabling you to manage stress and emotional triggers more effectively.

Think of the tightness in your chest when you're anxious or the knots in your stomach before a stressful meeting. These are your body's signals, offering a glimpse into what's going on beneath the surface. Through somatic practices, you learn to translate these signals into actionable insights, allowing you to move forward with a sense of wholeness.

The benefits of somatic therapy are both immediate and far-reaching. One of its key advantages is improved emotional regulation, as it teaches you to recognize and process physical sensations linked to your emotions. By addressing these sensations, somatic therapy can alleviate chronic pain and other physical symptoms often tied to unresolved trauma.

Beyond physical relief, it promotes effective stress management, helping lower stress levels and enhance overall well-being. Perhaps most importantly, somatic therapy deepens the mind–body connection, offering insight into how your physical and emotional states influence each other—creating a foundation for lasting healing.

Think of your mind and body as dance partners—sometimes they're perfectly in sync; other times, one steps on the other's toes! Somatic therapy helps them rediscover harmony.

In essence, somatic therapy offers a holistic approach to healing that bridges the gap between mind and body. It equips you with practical tools to address trauma, anxiety, and chronic pain—moving beyond traditional methods to embrace the interconnected nature of your physical and emotional health.

As you explore the principles and practices ahead, you'll discover how these techniques can become transformative allies on your journey of healing.

1.2 THE SCIENCE BEHIND THE MIND–BODY CONNECTION

The "mind-body connection" is more than just a wellness cliché. It's a deeply rooted biological reality, and understanding it can be a game-changer for your healing. The nervous system plays a crucial role in this connection. It is the body's communication network, transmitting signals between the brain and various parts of the body.

When you feel stressed, your nervous system releases stress hormones like cortisol, preparing your body to fight or flee. This response is helpful in short bursts, but chronic stress keeps your body in a constant state of alert, which can lead to a host of physical and emotional problems.

Imagine your nervous system as a smoke alarm—it's designed to detect danger and keep you safe. But after trauma, that alarm can become overly sensitive, going off even when there's no threat. Trauma traps your body in a heightened state of "fight, flight, or freeze," even long after the danger has passed.

This is where somatic practices come in.

Healing isn't just about *thinking* your way through recovery—it requires your body to feel safe. Practices like breathwork, yoga, and grounding directly engage your body's calming systems, helping to reset your nervous system and create the conditions needed for emotional recovery.

Polyvagal Theory, developed by neuroscientist Stephen Porges, sheds light on how our nervous system responds to stress and trauma. According to this theory, the vagus nerve—a fundamental part of the parasympathetic nervous system—regulates our emotional and physiological states. You can think of the vagus nerve as the body's emotional dimmer switch, helping you adjust between calm, action, and shutdown states. When you experience trauma, your body can get stuck in either a hyper-aroused state (sympathetic) or a shutdown state (dorsal vagal). Somatic therapy uses techniques to stimulate the vagus nerve, helping to restore balance and emotional regulation.

Neuroplasticity, the brain's adaptability, is another fascinating concept that plays a role in the mind–body connection. It refers to the brain's ability to reorganize itself by forming new neural connections throughout life. Neuroplasticity works like a path through a forest— the more you walk a new path, the clearer it becomes, until it eventually replaces the old route. Trauma can disrupt these connections, but the good news is that the brain can adapt.

Through repeated, small changes, somatic therapy can help create new, healthy neural pathways. For instance, practicing mindfulness or engaging in gentle movement like yoga can help rewire the brain, promoting healing and emotional resilience. Understanding these physiological principles will deepen your appreciation of how somatic therapy can transform body and mind.

Scientific evidence supporting somatic therapy is robust and growing. A study published in the journal *Traumatology* found that somatic experiencing significantly reduced PTSD symptoms in participants. Another research review highlighted the effectiveness of eye movement desensitization and reprocessing (EMDR), a form of somatic therapy, in treating emotional trauma. These evidence-based practices have shown high success rates in both clinical settings and real-world applications, making somatic therapy a reliable option for those seeking relief from trauma and stress.

Stress and trauma don't just affect the mind; they leave a mark on the body as well. Chronic stress can lead to conditions like high blood pressure and digestive issues. When you experience trauma, your body goes into survival mode. This response might involve tightening muscles, shallow breathing, or a racing heart. Over time, if these reactions become habitual, they can lead to long-term health issues. Unresolved trauma can manifest as chronic pain, fibromyalgia, or other stress-related illnesses, making it crucial to address both the emotional and physical aspects of healing. The body doesn't forget trauma—it stores it like muscle memory, waiting for the right tools to release and heal.

Somatic therapy offers powerful techniques for releasing tension and trauma stored in the body. One standard method, "pendulation," involves moving between feelings of safety and discomfort to gradually release stored energy. Another technique, "titration," helps you feel physical sensations in small, manageable increments, preventing overwhelm. These methods work to rewire the nervous system, promoting resilience and restoring balance. By focusing on body awareness and mindful movement, somatic therapy can help you break free from the grip of chronic stress and trauma.

Imagine sitting at your desk, feeling the familiar tension in your shoulders. You take a moment to close your eyes and focus on your breath. As you breathe deeply, you notice the tightness beginning to ease. This one simple act of awareness and intentional breathing is a small example of how somatic therapy works.

Over time, these practices can significantly improve your physical and emotional health, helping you navigate life's challenges with greater ease and resilience.

In essence, the science behind the mind–body connection provides a solid foundation for the effectiveness of somatic therapy. By understanding how our nervous system, brain, and body interact, we can better appreciate the transformative power of these practices. Whether you're dealing with the aftermath of trauma, or the daily grind of chronic stress, somatic therapy offers a path toward healing that is both grounded in science—and deeply compassionate.

1.3 KEY CONCEPTS: GROUNDING, BODY AWARENESS, AND SELF-REGULATION

Grounding is a fundamental concept in somatic therapy. Grounding is like anchoring a ship—it keeps you steady, even when the waves of life get choppy. Imagine having a stressful day at work, your mind racing with deadlines and tasks. Grounding techniques help you pull your focus back to the present moment, anchoring you in the here and now.

One simple grounding exercise involves focusing on your breath. Sit comfortably, close your eyes, and take a deep breath through your nose, feeling your lungs expand. Exhale slowly through your mouth, letting go of any tension. Another effective technique is to feel your feet on the ground. Whether you're standing or sitting, take a moment to notice the sensation of your feet contacting the floor. These simple exercises can reduce anxiety and help you stay present, making it easier to manage stress and emotional overwhelm.

Body awareness is another cornerstone of somatic therapy. Developing this awareness involves tuning into the physical sensations in your body. One effective method is the body scan exercise. Start by finding a quiet place where you won't be disturbed. Lie down or sit comfortably and close your eyes. Begin by focusing on your toes, noticing any sensations without judgment. Gradually move your attention up through your body—feet, legs, hips, abdomen, chest, arms, and head. Pay attention to areas of tension or discomfort and simply observe them.

This practice increases sensitivity to bodily sensations and plays a crucial role in emotional regulation. By becoming more attuned to your body, you can recognize when you're feeling stressed or anxious and take steps to address these emotions before they escalate.

Self-regulation is the ability to manage your emotional responses and is vital for dealing with trauma and stress. Think of self-regulation like learning to drive a car smoothly—you're learning how to accelerate, brake, and navigate life's curves with more control and less wear and tear on your emotional engine.

Self-regulation techniques can help you maintain emotional equilibrium when faced with a stressful situation. Breathwork is a powerful tool for this. For example, the 4-7-8 breathing technique involves inhaling through your nose for a count of four, holding your breath for a count of seven, and exhaling through your mouth for a count of eight.

Progressive muscle relaxation is another helpful technique. Starting with your toes, tense each muscle group for a few seconds before releasing the tension. Move up through your body, finishing with your head and neck.

To bring these concepts into your daily life, let's explore some practical exercises. A daily grounding routine can be as simple as spending five minutes each morning focusing on your breath and feeling your feet on the ground. Guided body awareness meditations can be integrated into your evening routine, helping you unwind and reflect on the day.

For self-regulation, consider setting aside time during your lunch break to practice breathwork. If you find yourself in a particularly stressful situation, such as a heated meeting or a crowded commute, use progressive muscle relaxation to calm your mind and body.

During a long day at work, use body awareness techniques to check in with yourself periodically, noticing and addressing any tension areas. If you're dealing with a difficult conversation, take a moment to ground yourself by focusing on your breath before responding. If you're overwhelmed by emotions, self-regulation techniques like breathwork and progressive muscle relaxation can help you regain control and composure.

Grounding, body awareness, and self-regulation are practical tools you can use daily. These practices form the foundation of somatic therapy, offering an accessible and effective pathway to healing.

As you continue to explore these techniques, they will become second nature, empowering you to manage stress and trauma increasingly more effectively.

1.4 TRAUMA-INFORMED APPROACH: SAFE AND SUPPORTIVE PRACTICES

Imagine creating a space where you instantly feel safe and supported. The lighting is soft, the atmosphere is calming, and you know you're in a place where you can let your guard down. This type of environment is crucial when practicing trauma-informed care. Just as a trauma-informed therapist would guide you through healing with care and respect, it's essential to extend the same kindness to yourself as you explore these practices on your own.

A trauma-informed approach is like learning to swim in shallow water first—it ensures you feel safe and supported before diving into deeper emotional currents.

Safety, trustworthiness, and empowerment are the three foundational principles that guide trauma-informed. These elements form the foundation for creating a space where healing can occur without the risk of re-traumatization.

- Safety is the first and most essential principle. When healing from trauma, it's non-negotiable to feel physically and emotionally safe in your environment.

- Trustworthiness is about being transparent and consistent with yourself. Self-care requires building trust in your process and being honest about your boundaries and capacities.
- Empowerment involves giving yourself the tools and confidence to take control of your healing journey. You are responsible for setting your pace and deciding which practices resonate with you. These principles work together to create a personal space where you can explore and heal from your trauma without fear.

Re-traumatization is a risk even when working through self-care. It occurs when certain activities or experiences inadvertently trigger a traumatic response. Establishing clear boundaries and giving yourself permission to stop, adjust, or modify any self-care practice that feels overwhelming is essential. You may try something different or take a break if an activity begins to feel triggering. The goal is to foster an environment where you feel heard, validated, and respected—by yourself—*no matter what* emotions or memories surface.

Building self-trust is another crucial aspect of trauma-informed self-care. Trust doesn't happen overnight; it takes time, consistency, and self-compassion. Take time to know your needs, listen to your body's signals, and respect your personal boundaries.

Techniques like active self-reflection, self-empathy, and consistent self-support can help create a solid foundation of trust. As this trust develops, you will feel more comfortable and open, making it easier to explore and address trauma on your terms.

One helpful somatic therapy model is the Window of Tolerance, developed by Dr. Dan Siegel. This model describes the optimal zone where you can function effectively and feel emotionally regulated. You can think clearly, manage your emotions, and respond appropriately to stress within your window.

However, when you're *outside* your window, you may become either hyper-aroused (anxious, overwhelmed) or hypo-aroused (numb, disconnected). Trauma-informed self-care aims to help you stay within your window of tolerance, where healing can occur.

When you start feeling overwhelmed, grounding techniques—such as focusing on your breath or the sensation of your feet on the ground—can help bring you back to the present moment. Self-regulation practices, such as breathwork or progressive muscle relaxation, can help you manage your emotional responses and stay within your window of tolerance. Integrating these strategies into daily life will help you manage stress and emotional triggers.

Handling emotional responses during your self-care process can be challenging. Strong emotions often surface when you're dealing with trauma, and it's crucial to have strategies in place to manage these reactions. Grounding and calming techniques can be incredibly beneficial in these moments.

For example, taking slow, deep breaths or focusing on a comforting object can help you stay grounded when emotions rise. Methods for processing and integrating emotional experiences are also crucial. You might find it helpful to express your feelings through journaling, art, or movement, to process your emotions.

Self-care practices after an intense session are essential for maintaining your well-being. After a particularly emotional experience, it's imperative to decompress and care for yourself. Consider taking a warm bath, walking in nature, or engaging in a relaxing activity you enjoy. Developing a post-care routine that includes grounding and calming techniques can help you transition from your self-care practice to your daily life.

Creating a trauma-informed, safe, and supportive environment is not just about following a set of guidelines; it's about genuinely caring for your well-being. Every step ensures you feel safe, supported, and empowered throughout your healing process.

Healing from trauma is a deeply personal experience that requires sensitivity, patience, and understanding. Just as every seed needs the right conditions to grow, healing begins with small, intentional steps. The principles and practices you'll explore in the following chapters are here to help you cultivate that growth, one moment at a time.

Before moving on, take a moment for reflection.

Reflection Prompt: Recognizing Your Starting Point

As you begin the journey of reading this book, take a moment to reflect on where you are right now.

What emotions, physical sensations, or thoughts are most present for you?

How does your body feel at this moment?

Write down any challenges you face and what you hope to achieve through this healing process.

This reflection will help you recognize your starting point and provide insight as you move forward.

2

EMOTIONAL AND PHYSICAL HEALING TECHNIQUES

Stress can hit us hard, making it difficult to think clearly—or even breathe sometimes. I remember one chaotic day: the kids were restless, meals weren't going as planned, and I was drowning in tasks and also emotions. At a certain moment, I remembered to breathe— and everything changed. I took a few minutes to focus solely on my breathing, inhaling deeply and exhaling slowly. I was amazed at how quickly my mind and body began to calm down. Before this breathwork, my thoughts were racing, and I felt my heart pounding. But as I breathed deeply, the tension in my shoulders eased, and a sense of calm washed over me.

This first part of the chapter discusses how you can harness the power of breathwork for emotional regulation.

2.1 BREATHWORK FOR EMOTIONAL REGULATION

Breathwork, or controlled breathing, is a simple yet effective way to manage your emotions and calm your nervous system. When you're stressed, your body releases stress hormones. Breathwork helps reduce these hormones, bringing your body back to a state of balance.

Deep breathing stimulates the vagus nerve, which activates the parasympathetic nervous system—your body's natural "rest and digest" mode. This process calms you down and enhances your overall health and vitality.

One of the most straightforward techniques in breathwork is diaphragmatic breathing, also known as "belly breathing". This method helps you take fuller, deeper breaths, reducing tension and promoting relaxation. To practice diaphragmatic breathing:

1. Sit or lie down in a comfortable position.
2. Place one hand on your chest and the other on your belly.
3. Inhale deeply through your nose, allowing your belly to rise while keeping your chest relatively still.
4. Exhale slowly through your mouth, letting your belly fall.
5. Repeat this for a few minutes, and you'll notice a significant decrease in stress and anxiety.

Another effective technique is box breathing, which is excellent for stress reduction. Box breathing involves inhaling, holding, exhaling, and pausing for equal counts. To try this, sit comfortably and close your eyes. Inhale deeply for a count of four, hold for four, exhale slowly for four, and pause again for four. Repeat this pattern several times. By slowing your breath in a steady rhythm, box breathing helps calm the nervous system and sharpen focus.

For balance and mental clarity, alternate nostril breathing is an effective practice. This technique involves breathing through one nostril at a time, which can help balance your brain's left and right hemispheres. To practice this:

1. Sit comfortably and close your eyes.
2. Use your right thumb to close your right nostril, and inhale deeply through your left nostril.
3. Close your left nostril with your right ring finger and release your right nostril.

4. Exhale through your right nostril.
5. Inhale through your right nostril, close it with your thumb, and exhale through your left nostril.
6. Continue this pattern for several minutes.

Alternate nostril breathing can leave you feeling balanced and refreshed.

The 4-7-8 breathing technique is particularly effective for anxiety relief. This method involves inhaling for four seconds, holding the breath for seven seconds, and exhaling for eight seconds. To practice:

1. Sit or lie down comfortably.
2. Close your eyes and inhale through your nose for a count of four.
3. Hold your breath for a count of seven.
4. Exhale through your mouth for a count of eight.
5. Repeat this cycle three to four times.

The 4-7-8 technique helps slow down your heart rate and promotes a sense of calm.

Integrating breathwork into your daily routine is easier than you might think. Start your day with a few minutes of diaphragmatic breathing to set a calm tone. Take short breaks to practice box breathing throughout the day, especially during stressful moments. Incorporate alternate nostril breathing into your evening routine to balance your energy before bed. Combining breathwork with other somatic practices, like yoga or mindfulness meditation, can enhance its benefits. For example, you might start a yoga session with a few rounds of 4-7-8 breathing to center yourself.

Incorporating these techniques into your life will make a significant difference to your quality of life. Imagine starting your day with a sense of calm, tackling work with focused energy, and winding down in the evening with a clear mind.

Breathwork is just one way to regulate your emotions, but mindful movement offers another powerful avenue for healing. Let's explore how yoga can enhance both emotional and physical well-being.

2.2 MOVEMENT PRACTICES: YOGA FOR EMOTIONAL AND PHYSICAL HEALING

Yoga has a special place in somatic therapy. It's not just about stretching or achieving a perfect pose; it's about tuning into your body and mind. Yoga deepens body awareness, helping you tune into the signals your body sends. This heightened awareness plays a significant role in emotional regulation.

The combination of mindful movement and breathwork calms the nervous system, lowering stress hormones and promoting relaxation. Additionally, yoga enhances flexibility and strength, making your body more resilient to physical and emotional stress.

Certain yoga poses are particularly effective for emotional regulation. **Child's Pose**, for instance, is a grounding pose that helps you feel safe and secure. To practice Child's Pose, kneel on the floor, touch your big toes together, and sit back on your heels. Spread your knees wide apart and lay your torso down between your thighs. Extend your arms forward with palms facing down.

Rest your forehead on the mat and breathe deeply.

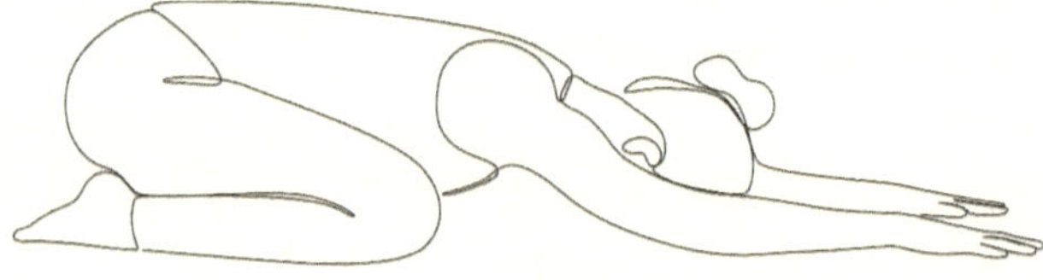

Child's pose can help calm your mind and bring you back to the present moment.

Warrior II is another powerful pose, especially for building confidence. Stand with your feet wide apart, about three to four feet. Turn your right foot out 90 degrees and your left foot slightly in. Extend your arms out to the sides at shoulder height, palms facing down. Bend your right knee, making sure it's directly over your ankle. Gaze over your right hand and hold the pose.

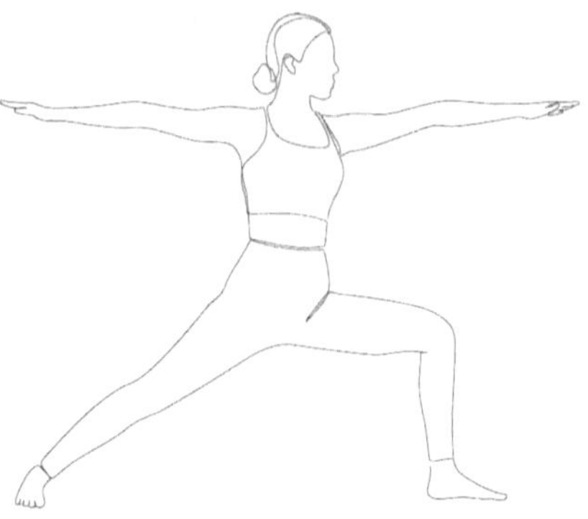

Warrior II strengthens your legs and core, while boosting your confidence and focus.

For relaxation, **Legs-Up-The-Wall** is excellent. Sit sideways next to a wall and swing your legs up as you lie back, bringing your hips as close to the wall as possible. Rest your arms by your sides with palms facing up. Close your eyes and breathe deeply.

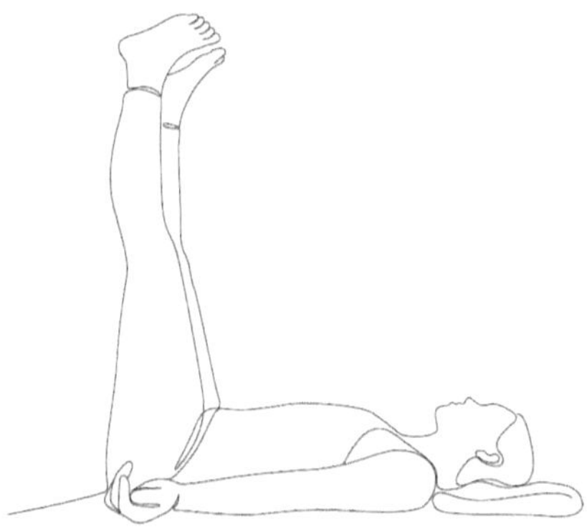

This pose helps reduce stress and anxiety by promoting blood circulation and calming the nervous system.

Corpse Pose, or Savasana, is the ultimate pose for complete release. Lie flat on your back, legs extended, arms resting by your sides, and palms facing up. Close your eyes and let your body relax completely. Focus on your breath and let go of any tension.

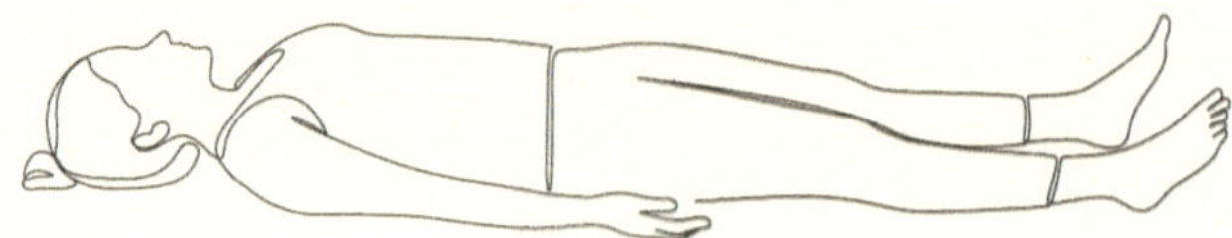

Savasana allows your body and mind to rest deeply, promoting relaxation and emotional release.

Cat-Cow is a dynamic sequence that promotes spinal flexibility and emotional release. Start on your hands and knees in a tabletop position. Inhale as you arch your back, lifting your head and tailbone towards the ceiling (Cow Pose). Exhale as you round your spine, tucking your chin to your chest and drawing your belly button towards your spine (Cat Pose).

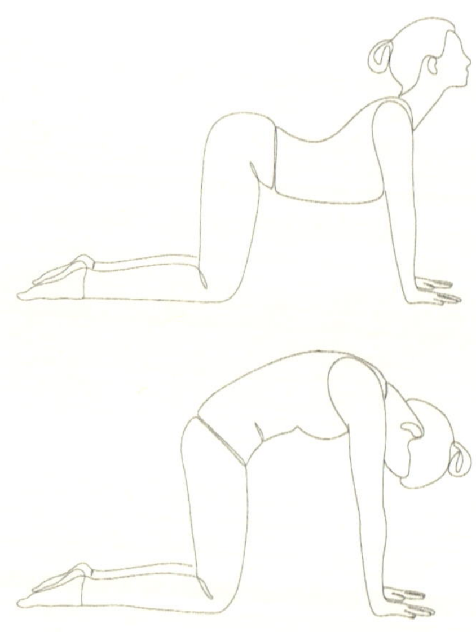

Repeat this sequence several times, moving with your breath. Cat-Cow helps release tension in your spine and can have a soothing effect on your emotions.

These poses are accessible to all, regardless of experience level. For Child's Pose, if you have knee discomfort, place a blanket or bolster between your thighs and calves for added support. In Warrior II, if balance is an issue, position yourself near a wall for added stability. Place a cushion under your hips if your hamstrings are tight for Legs-Up-The-Wall. Use a rolled-up blanket under your knees in Savasana to relieve lower back tension. During Cat-Cow, if you have sensitive wrists, perform the sequence on your forearms instead of your hands.

Always listen to your body and modify poses as needed.

Let's discuss yoga sequences tailored to specific issues. For anxiety relief, a calming evening sequence can work wonders. Start with Child's Pose to ground yourself, then move into Legs-Up-The-Wall for relaxation. Follow with a few rounds of Cat-Cow to release tension in your spine. End with Savasana, allowing your body to rest completely. This sequence can help calm your mind and prepare you for a restful night's sleep.

An energizing morning flow can set a positive tone for the day and help manage PTSD. Begin with Warrior II to build confidence and strength—transition into Cat-Cow to promote spinal flexibility and release stored tension. Finish with Legs-Up-The-Wall to balance your energy. This sequence can help you start your day with empowerment and resilience.

If you're dealing with chronic pain, a gentle yoga sequence can provide relief. Start with Legs-Up-The-Wall to promote blood circulation and reduce tension. Move into Child's Pose for grounding and gentle stretching. Follow with Cat-Cow to release tension in your spine. End with Savasana, allowing your body to relax completely.

Yoga is a way to connect with yourself on a deeper level. It's not about perfection—it's about being present with yourself. Every stretch and every breath are steps toward greater peace and self-connection.

While yoga focuses on mindful movement, Tai Chi offers another gentle way to connect body and mind. Let's explore how this ancient practice can reduce stress and enhance body awareness.

2.3 TAI CHI FOR STRESS REDUCTION AND BODY AWARENESS

Imagine waking up one morning and feeling balanced and calm throughout the day. That's the magic of Tai Chi. Originating in ancient China, Tai Chi is both a martial art and a form of meditative movement. Its history spans centuries, blending physical postures with breath coordination and mindfulness. The practice is based on principles emphasizing slow, deliberate movements synchronized with deep, rhythmic breathing and a focused mind. This combination makes Tai Chi an excellent inclusion in somatic therapy, offering a holistic emotional and physical wellness approach.

One of the most significant benefits of Tai Chi is its ability to enhance balance and coordination. The slow, flowing movements require you to be fully present, paying attention to how your body moves through space. Additionally, Tai Chi is a powerful tool for reducing stress and anxiety. The mindful movements and deep breathing techniques activate the parasympathetic nervous system, promoting relaxation and reducing the production of stress hormones.

Another benefit of Tai Chi is its ability to improve body awareness and mindfulness. As you move through the different postures, you become more attuned to your body's sensations. This heightened awareness helps you recognize areas of tension or discomfort, allowing you to address these issues before they escalate. Moreover, the meditative aspect of Tai Chi encourages a state of mindfulness, where you focus on the present moment, rather than worrying about the past or future.

Let's explore some basic Tai Chi movements you can easily try at home. One of the most accessible movements is the "wave hands like clouds" sequence. Start by standing with your feet shoulder-width apart and knees slightly bent. Raise your arms to chest level, with your palms facing down. Shift your weight to your right foot, gently turning your torso to the right as your left hand glides across your body. Now shift to your left foot, twisting your torso to the left and allowing your right hand to float across your body. Repeat this fluid, wave-like movement for several minutes, focusing on your breath and the fluidity of your movements.

Try a sequence that includes grounding and centering movements for a simple morning practice. Begin with the "wave hands like clouds" sequence to warm up and enter the flow. Next, move into the "parting the wild horse's mane" posture. Stand with your feet shoulder-width apart, knees slightly bent. Raise your arms to chest level, with your right hand in front of your chest and your left hand below it, palms facing each other. Step forward with your left foot, shifting your weight onto it as you push your right hand forward and pull your left hand back, as if parting a horse's mane. Repeat on the other side, stepping forward with your right foot and switching the positions of your hands. This sequence helps ground you and center your energy, preparing you for the day ahead.

To incorporate Tai Chi into your daily life, start with short daily routines to build the habit. Dedicate 10–15 minutes each morning or evening to practice a simple sequence. Combining Tai Chi with breathwork and meditation can enhance its benefits. For example, begin your Tai Chi practice with a few minutes of deep breathing to center yourself, move through your chosen sequence, and end with a brief meditation to solidify the calmness.

Using Tai Chi as a mindful break during the day can also be incredibly beneficial. Whenever you feel stressed or overwhelmed, take a few minutes to practice a simple Tai Chi movement, bringing you back to a state of balance and calm.

Tai Chi offers a gentle yet powerful way to reduce stress and enhance body awareness. Its slow, mindful movements and deep breathing techniques make it an ideal practice for anyone looking to integrate somatic therapy into their daily life. By starting with basic movements and gradually building up your practice, you can experience the many benefits of Tai Chi.

For visual demonstrations of "wave hands like clouds" and "parting the wild horse's mane," I recommend looking for instructional videos by certified Tai Chi instructors. YouTube has many helpful resources —try searching for "Tai Chi Wave Hands Like Clouds tutorial" or "Tai Chi Parting the Wild Horse's Mane tutorial." To ensure accurate and safe guidance, look for videos from experienced practitioners or reputable organizations, such as the Tai Chi for Health Institute.

2.4 PILATES FOR STRENGTHENING THE MIND-BODY CONNECTION

Much like yoga and Tai Chi, Pilates offers a unique way to enhance the mind-body connection. At its core, Pilates focuses on control, concentration, and centering. These principles guide every movement, ensuring your mind fully engages with your body. Control involves performing exercises with precision, avoiding any jerky or rushed movements. Concentration entails directing your full attention to each movement while noticing how your body feels and responds. Centering focuses on engaging your core muscles, which Pilates often refers to as the "powerhouse." Engaging your core strengthens your body and helps you stay grounded and balanced.

Emotionally, Pilates can be incredibly grounding. Focusing on controlled movements and deep breathing can calm your mind and reduce stress. Physically, Pilates improves flexibility, strength, and posture, making your body more resilient. It also promotes better body awareness, helping you tune into your body's subtle signals. This heightened awareness can be especially beneficial for emotional regulation, as it allows you to recognize and address stress or anxiety before it intensifies.

Let's introduce some essential Pilates exercises that are particularly effective for emotional regulation. **The Hundred** is a classic Pilates exercise focusing on breath control and core strength.

To perform the Hundred:

1. Lie on your back with your legs lifted to a tabletop position and your arms by your sides.
2. Lift your head, neck, and shoulders off the mat, and extend your legs to a 45-degree angle.
3. Begin pumping your arms up and down while inhaling for five counts and exhaling for five counts.
4. Continue this pattern until you reach 100 pumps.

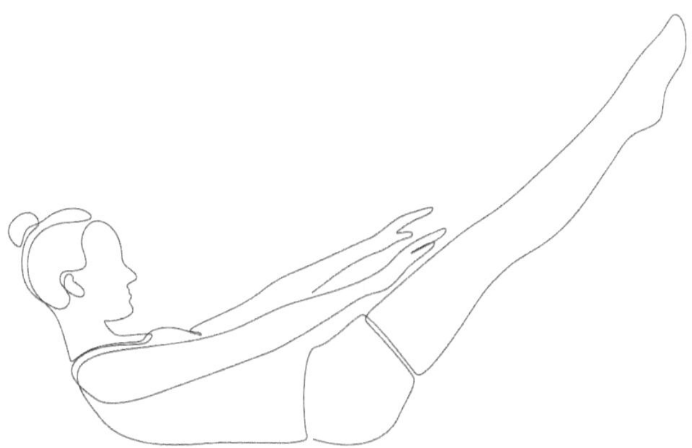

This exercise engages your core and promotes deep, rhythmic breathing, which calms your mind and body.

The Roll-Up is another excellent exercise for spinal flexibility and emotional release. Start by lying on your back with your arms extended overhead and legs straight.

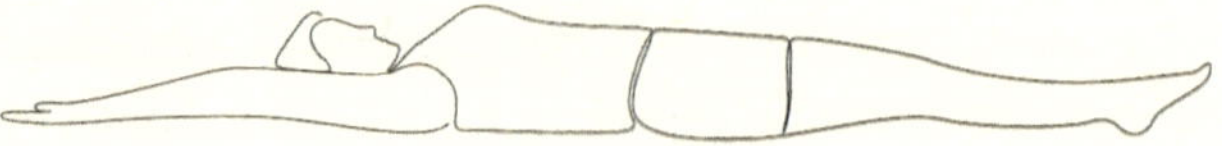

Inhale to prepare, then exhale as you slowly roll up, reaching your hands towards your toes.

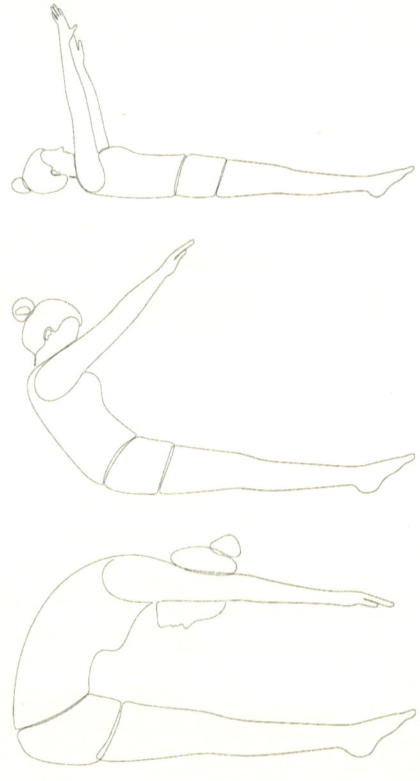

Inhale as you hold the stretch, then exhale as you slowly roll back down to the starting position. The Roll-Up stretches your spine and engages your core, helping to release tension and promote relaxation.

Single-Leg Circles are great for improving coordination and focus. Lie on your back with your legs straight. Lift your right leg towards the ceiling, keeping it straight. Begin making small circles with your leg, moving from the hip. Perform five circles in one direction, then switch to the opposite direction. Repeat with your left leg. This exercise engages your core and requires concentration, helping to center your mind and body.

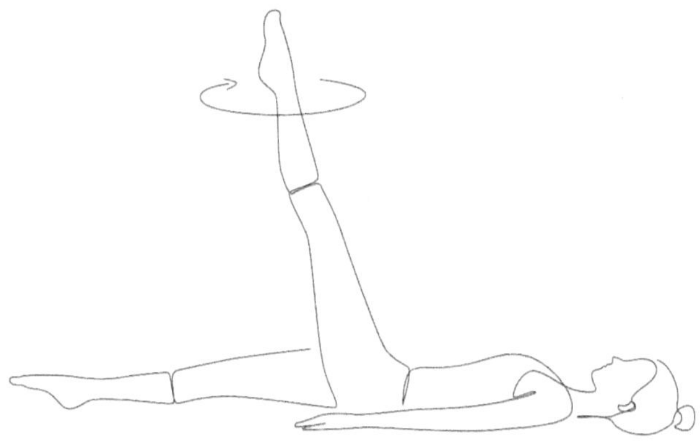

The Spine Stretch Forward is perfect for relaxation. Sit on the mat with your legs extended straight in front of you and your feet flexed. Extend your arms straight out in front of you at shoulder height. Inhale to prepare, then exhale as you reach forward, rounding your spine and bringing your head towards your knees. Hold the stretch for a few breaths, then inhale as you slowly return to the starting position. Stretching your spine while breathing deeply releases tension and calms your mind.

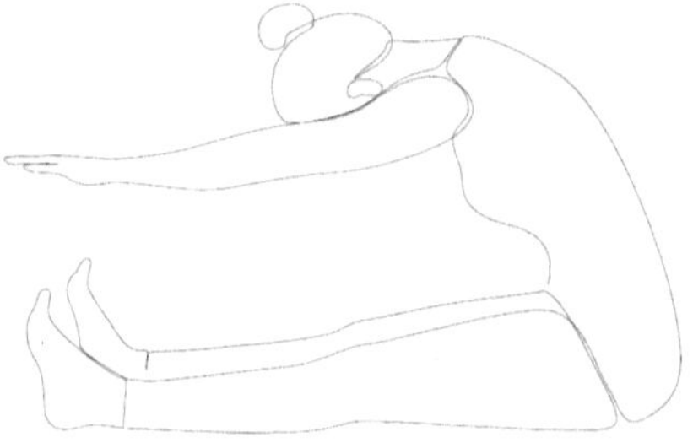

If lifting your legs to a 45-degree angle is too challenging for the Hundred, keep them bent at a tabletop position. If rolling all the way up is difficult during the Roll-Up, place your hands behind your thighs for support. For Single-Leg Circles, bend your knee slightly if keeping your leg straight is challenging. When performing the Spine Stretch Forward, if you can't reach your toes, place a cushion under your knees to make the stretch more comfortable. Always listen to your body and modify exercises as needed.

Pilates routines can be tailored to address specific issues like trauma, anxiety, and chronic pain. For chronic pain relief, a gentle routine can work wonders. Start with the Spine Stretch Forward to release tension in your back. Move into Single-Leg Circles to improve coordination and gently engage your core. Finish with the Hundred, keeping your legs bent to reduce strain.

For an energizing morning practice, start with the Hundred to wake up your core and get your blood flowing. Follow with the Roll-Up to stretch your spine and engage your entire body. End with Single-Leg Circles to improve coordination and focus. Performing this sequence can help you start your day feeling strong and centered.

In the evening, a calming routine can help you unwind. Begin with the Spine Stretch Forward to release tension from the day. Move into the Roll-Up to stretch your spine and promote relaxation. Finish with the Hundred, focusing on deep, rhythmic breathing to calm your mind and body. This routine can help you transition into a restful night's sleep.

Pilates builds strength and awareness over time. Every slight improvement brings you closer to a deeper mind-body connection. These practices—breathwork, yoga, Tai Chi, and Pilates—offer unique emotional and physical healing benefits. As you explore these techniques, remember: the goal isn't perfection but *progress*.

You'll build resilience and reconnect with yourself with small, intentional steps—one breath and one movement at a time.

Reflection Prompt: Emotional and Physical Healing Techniques

Take a moment to reflect on the practices introduced in this chapter and how they can integrate into your daily life:

- Which breathwork or movement technique resonated most with you? Why?
- How can you incorporate these practices during moments of stress or anxiety?
- What small step can you take today to integrate breathwork, yoga, Tai Chi, or Pilates into your routine?

Jot down your thoughts, and revisit this reflection regularly to track how these practices impact your emotional and physical well-being over time.

3

CUSTOMIZABLE HEALING PLANS

Designing your own personal somatic therapy plan is like tuning an instrument. Every practice is a string; harmony is created in your healing journey when each is appropriately tuned. This chapter is your guide to crafting a 28-day somatic therapy program tailored to your unique needs.

3.1 DESIGNING YOUR 28-DAY SOMATIC THERAPY PROGRAM

Let's start with the structure of your 28-day program. This simple yet effective framework is divided into weekly themes, with targeted exercises and periods for integration and reflection. Each week has a specific focus, drawing from concepts discussed in other parts of this book, allowing you to build on the skills and techniques you learn as you progress.

Week 1 focuses on grounding and body awareness—your foundation. Refer to Chapter 1 to practice techniques like grounding exercises and body scans to attune to physical sensations. These tools keep you present and connected to your body, preparing you for enhanced emotional work.

Week 2 focuses on emotional regulation, draws from breathwork and movement practices introduced in Chapter 2. These techniques are designed to help you manage your emotions effectively. Whether it's the 4-7-8 breathing method to calm anxiety or progressive muscle relaxation to release tension, this week provides tools to navigate emotional highs and lows.

In **Week 3**, you'll explore advanced somatic practices found in Chapter 7. This week is about deepening your skills and exploring more complex techniques. You might try somatic experiencing exercises to release stored trauma or advanced breathwork for more profound emotional healing. The goal is to build on your established foundation and enhance your somatic therapy toolkit.

Week 4 focuses on integration and resilience building, starting in Chapter 8. You'll reflect on your progress and integrate what you've learned into your daily life. You are engaging in practices that foster resilience to help you maintain the gains you've made. This week includes activities like reflective journaling, where you can document your experiences and insights, and resilience-building exercises to strengthen your emotional and physical well-being.

At the end of this chapter, you will find a worksheet for Week 1 of the 28-Day Program. This Daily Tracker comes with detailed instructions for working through each day of the week.

Customization is vital to making this program work for you. Think of this program as a recipe—while the ingredients are provided, feel free to adjust portions and seasonings to suit your taste. Choose preferred exercises and practices that resonate with you. If you find specific techniques more effective or enjoyable, incorporate them more frequently. Adjust the intensity and duration of exercises based on your comfort level and progress.

For instance, if you're new to breathwork, start with shorter sessions and gradually increase the duration as you become more comfortable.

Set personal goals and milestones to keep yourself motivated. Whether mastering a new technique or noticing a reduction in stress levels, these milestones provide a sense of accomplishment and encourage you to keep going.

Supporting materials and resources are important for enhancing your experience with somatic therapy. Throughout this book and program, you'll find journaling prompts designed to help you reflect on your journey and gain valuable insights into your progress.

Journaling Prompt: Reflection and Integration

Take a few minutes each day to reflect on your experiences. Use the following prompt to guide your journaling: "What sensations, emotions, or thoughts did I notice during today's practice? How did these experiences affect my overall well-being?" This reflection helps you stay connected to your process and track your progress over time. Are there practices that resonate with you or areas where you want to focus more deeply? Use these reflections to guide your choices as you fine-tune your personal healing plan.

This 28-day program is designed to be flexible, providing a clear path while allowing room for personalization. In the coming chapters, you'll explore additional tools—like mindfulness exercises, trauma-informed techniques, and heart rate variability biofeedback—which you can integrate into your 28-day program. Following the weekly themes can build a strong foundation, deepen your skills, and enable you to incorporate these practices into your life.

Imagine each day of this program as laying a single brick. By the end of 28 days, you'll have built a foundation to support your ongoing pursuit of balance.

3.2 DAILY 10-MINUTE PRACTICES FOR BUSY SCHEDULES

Finding time for self-care can feel impossible when life gets hectic. Yet, the benefits of daily practice, even if brief, can be transformative. Consistency is crucial. Building habits and routines helps you maintain progress and momentum. It's like watering a plant regularly; small, consistent efforts yield growth over time. Daily practices reduce stress, improve emotional regulation, and help you stay grounded. Integrating these practices into your routine will become second nature, making it easier to manage life's ups and downs.

Quick and effective practices can fit into any schedule. Let's start with a five-minute breathwork session. Find a quiet space and sit comfortably. Close your eyes and focus on your breath. Inhale deeply through your nose for a count of four, hold for seven, and exhale through your mouth for eight. Repeat this cycle for five minutes. This simple exercise calms your mind and body, reducing stress and anxiety.

Next, consider a quick body scan meditation. Sit or lie down in a comfortable position. Close your eyes and take a few deep breaths. Start by focusing on your toes and noticing any sensations. Gradually move your attention up through your body, from your feet to your head. Pay attention to areas of tension and simply observe them without judgment. This practice helps you become more aware of your body and can be done in just a few minutes.

A short yoga sequence can be incredibly effective for those moments when you need a physical reset. Begin with Child's Pose to ground yourself—transition into Cat-Cow to mobilize your spine and release tension. Finish with a few deep, mindful breathing rounds in Savasana (Corpse Pose) to relax completely. This sequence, which can be done in about 10 minutes, leaves you feeling refreshed and centered.

A brief Tai Chi movement is an excellent option if you prefer a more dynamic practice. Start with the "wave hands like clouds" sequence. Stand with your feet shoulder-width apart, knees slightly bent. Raise your arms to chest level, palms facing down. Shift your weight to your right foot as you turn your torso to the right, allowing your left hand to float across your body. Shift your weight to your left foot, twist your torso to the left, and let your right hand float across your body. Continue this gentle, wave-like motion for a few minutes. This practice promotes relaxation and improves body awareness.

Timing cues can make these practices easy to follow. Set a timer for the five-minute breathwork session and focus on your breath. With the body scan meditation, spend about 10–15 seconds on each body part, moving slowly up your body. For the yoga sequence, spend about two minutes in each pose, focusing on your breath and the sensations in your body. The Tai Chi movement can be done for about five minutes, allowing you to get into a flow without feeling rushed. These timing cues help maximize the effectiveness of each practice, even in a short amount of time.

Daily 10-minute practices are an essential part of your 28-day program. On especially hectic days, these brief sessions will help you stay on track and maintain momentum in your healing journey. Integrating these practices into your daily life doesn't have to be complicated. Start your morning with a quick body scan meditation or a five-minute breathwork session to set a calm tone for the day.

During midday breaks, a short yoga sequence or Tai Chi movement can help relieve stress and re-energize you. In the evening, wind down with a few minutes of breathwork or a body scan meditation to prepare for a restful night's sleep. Combining these practices with daily activities can make them more manageable. For example, you can practice mindful breathing while waiting for your coffee to brew, or do a quick body scan while lying in bed before sleep.

Consistency is key, but being flexible is also important. Life can be unpredictable. Feel free to choose from the various practices to adapt to different situations. The goal is to make these practices a regular, second-nature part of your routine, creating small pockets of calm and focus throughout your day. This consistency helps maintain progress and builds your resilience.

By integrating these 10-minute practices into your daily life, you can create a foundation of balance that will support you—no matter *how* busy your schedule gets. Remember, even small practices create meaningful shifts. Whether it's a quick breathwork session or a brief yoga stretch, these moments of self-care help you build resilience and bring a sense of calm to your day.

3.3 ADAPTING PRACTICES FOR DIFFERENT CONDITIONS: PTSD, ANXIETY, AND CHRONIC PAIN

Living with PTSD, anxiety, or chronic pain can feel like you are shouldering a heavy burden that never quite lifts. Each condition uniquely affects you, bringing its own set of challenges and symptoms. PTSD often manifests as flashbacks, nightmares, and hypervigilance. You might be easily startled or constantly on edge, which can be very exhausting.

Anxiety, on the other hand, comes with its own triggers and stressors. You may feel persistent worry or dread, even when there's no immediate threat. Common triggers can range from social situations to specific phobias, making everyday life feel overwhelming.

Chronic pain adds another layer of complexity, affecting both your physical and emotional well-being. The constant discomfort or pain can make it difficult to focus on anything else, leading to frustration and helplessness.

Given these unique needs, it's crucial to tailor your somatic practices to address each condition effectively. For PTSD, grounding techniques are particularly beneficial. These exercises help you stay connected to the present moment, reducing the intensity of flashbacks and dissociative episodes.

The 5-4-3-2-1 method uses your senses to anchor you in the present moment: Name five things you can see, four things you can touch, three sounds you can hear, two scents you can detect, and one thing you can taste. This technique can help anchor you in the present, making it easier to manage symptoms.

Breathwork can be a game-changer when it comes to managing anxiety. Techniques like box breathing or the 4-7-8 method can calm your nervous system and reduce anxiety levels. As mentioned earlier, box breathing involves inhaling for a count of four, holding your breath for four, exhaling for four, and holding again for four.

This method can help regulate your breath and bring a sense of calm. Alternatively, the 4-7-8 technique can be particularly effective in moments of acute anxiety, helping you regain control and focus.

Gentle movement is critical for those dealing with chronic pain. Practices like Tai Chi or gentle yoga can help alleviate physical discomfort and improve overall well-being. With its slow, flowing movements, Tai Chi can enhance body awareness and promote relaxation. Gentle yoga poses, like Child's Pose or Legs-Up-The-Wall, can also provide relief. These movements stretch and relax the muscles, reducing tension and pain.

Consider making some modifications as needed. Adjust the intensity and duration of exercises based on your comfort level. If you're new to breathwork, start with shorter sessions and gradually increase the time as you become more comfortable. Practice grounding techniques in a seated or lying-down position if standing is too challenging. Use props like cushions or blankets to support your body during yoga or Tai Chi.

These modifications can make the exercises more comfortable and efficient, allowing you to reap the benefits without overexerting yourself. The goal is to find what works best for you and incorporate it into your daily routine. Whether it's grounding exercises for PTSD, breathwork for anxiety, or gentle movement for chronic pain, these customized practices can significantly enhance your quality of life.

3.4 TRACKING PROGRESS AND ADJUSTING YOUR PLAN

Imagine starting a fitness routine without stepping on a scale or tracking your workouts. You'd have no idea if you were making progress, or if adjustments were needed. The same logic applies to your somatic therapy plan. Monitoring your progress is not just about celebrating milestones but about understanding patterns in your healing process. Tracking your progress during the 28-day program ensures you know your patterns and can adjust as needed. Use journaling prompts and progress logs to reflect on what's working—and what isn't. Recognizing these patterns ensures you stay motivated and on the right path. Every small achievement builds a sense of accomplishment that fuels further progress.

Growth requires flexibility. If some exercises become too easy, try increasing their intensity or exploring new techniques. On the other hand, if a practice feels overwhelming, it's okay to dial it back.

The key is finding a balance that works for you.

Diversifying your routine with new elements—like integrating Tai Chi or yoga with breathwork—prevents burnout and keeps things engaging.

Regular check-ins are essential to ensure your plan evolves with your needs. Use weekly assessments to make minor course corrections, asking:

Journaling Prompt: Weekly Check-In

Reflect on your progress at the end of each week. Use this weekly check-in as part of your 28-day program. Each week, evaluate which practices feel most supportive and whether you need to adjust your plan.

- What went well this week? What challenges did I face? What noticeable changes did I experience in my physical sensations or emotional state?

The Nonlinear Path of Healing

Tracking your progress isn't about rigidly following a plan but staying attuned to your evolving needs. Healing is not a straight path—it's okay to experience ups and downs along the way. Thoughtful adjustments ensure your somatic therapy plan remains both impactful and supportive.

Celebrate the Small Victories

Progress isn't always about remarkable milestones—the small victories along the way matter most. Every moment of awareness, each step forward, is a sign of growth. Celebrate these moments, no matter how small—they are the building blocks of resilience and well-being.

Crafting your healing plan is like tuning an instrument—it requires care, patience, and modest adjustments. Some strings may need tightening, others loosening, but every change brings you closer to harmony. With time, your chosen practices will align, creating a healing symphony unique to you.

Reflection Prompt: Tuning Your Healing Journey

As you begin crafting your personalized 28-day program, take a moment to reflect: What practices or activities resonate with you the most? Are there any goals you'd like to achieve through this plan—emotional, physical, or both? As your healing journey unfolds, return to these reflections to see how your needs evolve over time.

Instructions for Week 1 Daily Tracker: Grounding and Awareness

Welcome to Week 1 of your 28-Day Program!

This week, we focus on grounding exercises, body awareness, breathwork, and self-regulation—essential practices for reconnecting with your body, managing stress, and beginning to release stored tension.

How to Use Your Week 1 Tracker:

- **Daily Practice Focus**: Each day features a specific focus, such as body scanning, breathwork, or gentle movement. Before starting, read the practice description and consider how it aligns with your needs. Feel free to adapt each practice to suit what feels best for you. Refer to Chapter 1 for additional options or techniques.
- **Physical Sensations & Emotional State**: Track the physical sensations you notice during each practice. Are you feeling tension, relaxation, warmth, or something else? Reflect on your emotional state before and after each practice—did it help you feel calmer or more connected?
- **Challenges or Insights**: Record any challenges you faced or insights you gained. Was it difficult to focus, or did you experience new feelings of relaxation? Note any observations or realizations.
- **Daily Goal/Intention**: Set a simple goal or intention for each day, such as "remain present during the practice" or "approach with curiosity." This helps keep you focused and motivated.

Daily Practices for Week 1:

- **Day 1: Body Scan & Grounding Exercises**: Start with a body scan to tune into your sensations. Sit or lie down comfortably, bringing attention to each part of your body, starting from your toes. Follow with a grounding exercise, like feeling your feet on the ground or focusing on your breath.
- **Day 2: Progressive Muscle Relaxation**: Start at your toes and work your way up, paying attention as you release tension. Notice how releasing physical tension affects emotional stress.
- **Day 3: Diaphragmatic Breathing**: Place one hand on your belly and one on your chest. Inhale deeply through your nose, letting your belly rise, then exhale slowly through your mouth. This practice activates the body's relaxation response.
- **Day 4: Grounding with Gentle Movement**: Practice gentle stretching—reach your arms overhead, roll your shoulders, or stretch your neck. Notice how movement helps you reconnect with your body. If stretching doesn't feel right, try another grounding exercise from Chapter 1.
- **Day 5: Body Awareness Meditation**: Sit or lie quietly, bringing attention to different parts of your body. Observe sensations without judgment. This practice deepens your body connection and supports emotional regulation.
- **Day 6: Reflection & Integration**: Reflect on what you've learned and how the practices have impacted you. Write down key insights, growth moments, or areas where you feel more connected.
- **Day 7: Explore a Different Practice**: Revisit a practice from earlier in the week or try a different variation of grounding, body awareness, or self-regulation. Reflect on how it made you feel—did it deepen your connection to your body? Or help you feel more present?

Week 1 Daily Tracker: Grounding & Body Awareness

Day	Practice Focus	Physical Sensations	Emotional State	Challenges / Insights	Daily Goal / Intention
1	Body Scan & Grounding Exercises				
2	Progressive Muscle Relaxation				
3	Diaphragmatic Breathing				
4	Grounding with Gentle Movement (e.g., Gentle Stretching)				
5	Body Awareness Meditation				
6	Reflection & Integration				
7	Explore a Different Practice: Grounding, Body Awareness, or Self-Regulation				

4

MINDFULNESS TECHNIQUES AND EMOTIONAL RESILIENCE

One evening, my thoughts spiraled—bills to pay, deadlines looming, personal obligations—everything was piling up. It felt like I was drowning. In that moment of overwhelm, I remembered a simple practice: mindful breathing. I closed my eyes, inhaled deeply, and slowly exhaled. With each breath, I felt more grounded, more in control. The clarity of that moment illustrated the transformative power of mindfulness.

4.1 INTRODUCTION TO MINDFULNESS: CONCEPTS AND BENEFITS

Mindfulness means being fully present in the moment, aware of where you are and what you're doing, without being overly reactive or overwhelmed by what's happening around you. It's about tuning in to your experience without judgment, noticing your thoughts and feelings as they arise, and accepting them without trying to change or judge them.

Imagine sitting quietly and observing clouds drifting across the sky. Just as you wouldn't try to control the clouds, you don't attempt to control your thoughts or emotions; you simply let them pass.

The benefits of mindfulness are extensive and impactful. One of the most significant advantages is its ability to reduce stress and anxiety. When you practice mindfulness, you engage the parasympathetic nervous system, which helps your body relax and lowers stress hormones like cortisol. These techniques can lead to a noticeable decrease in anxiety and an overall sense of calm.

Mindfulness also enhances emotional regulation. By becoming more aware of your emotions, you can respond effectively rather than impulsively. Managing emotions leads to improved relationships and a more balanced life.

Mindfulness can also improve focus and concentration. When you practice being present, you train your brain to stay on task and resist distractions. This awareness can lead to better performance at work or school and a greater sense of accomplishment. Moreover, mindfulness strengthens the mind-body connection. By paying attention to bodily sensations, you become more attuned to your physical needs and can address them more promptly.

This heightened awareness can lead to better physical health and a greater sense of balanced health.

The science behind mindfulness is compelling. Research has proven that it can have profound effects on both mental and physical health. A study published in the journal, *Mindfulness* found that mindfulness practices can significantly reduce symptoms of depression and anxiety. Another study, conducted by Harvard researchers Benjamin Shapero and Gaëlle Desbordes, used functional magnetic resonance imaging (fMRI) to study the effects of mindfulness meditation on the brain. Their research indicated that changes in brain activity due to meditation persist even when individuals are *not* meditating, indicating long-term benefits. Neuroplasticity, the brain's ability to reorganize itself, is also enhanced by mindfulness practices, leading to lasting positive changes in brain structure and function.

Let's explore some basic mindfulness practices you can incorporate into your daily routine. Mindful breathing exercises are a great place to begin.

Find a quiet space and sit comfortably. Close your eyes and take a deep breath through your nose, feeling your lungs expand. Exhale slowly through your mouth, letting go of any tension. Focus on the sensations of your breath, noticing how it feels as it enters and leaves your body. If your mind wanders, gently bring your attention back to your breath. This simple practice can help calm your mind and reduce stress.

Another effective practice is observing your thoughts without judgment. Sit quietly and close your eyes. As thoughts arise, notice them without getting caught up in them. Imagine each thought as a leaf floating down a stream. Watch the leaf float by, and then let it go. This practice helps you develop a non-judgmental awareness of your thoughts, reducing the tendency to get stuck in negative thinking patterns.

Mindful eating is another powerful practice. The next time you eat, take a moment to be fully aware of your food. Look at the colors and textures, smell the aroma, and slowly taste each bite. Pay attention to the sensations in your mouth and the act of chewing and swallowing. This practice enhances your enjoyment of food and helps you become more aware of your body's hunger and fullness cues, promoting healthier eating habits.

The beauty of mindfulness lies in its simplicity and accessibility. You don't need any special equipment or much time to start experiencing its benefits. By incorporating these basic practices into your daily routine, you cultivate a greater sense of presence and reduce stress. Whether you're dealing with the pressures of daily life or seeking a deeper connection with yourself, mindfulness offers a powerful and effective path to healing and resilience.

Incorporate the mindfulness practices introduced here into your 28-day program. Use them during Week 1 as grounding tools, or revisit them during Week 4 to strengthen emotional resilience.

Reflection Prompt: Mindful Moments

At the end of each day, take a moment to reflect on any mindful experiences. Use this prompt to guide your journaling: *'What moments today did I feel most present and aware? How did these moments affect my emotional health?"*

Use this reflection throughout your 28-day program to stay connected with your mindfulness practice. Tracking these mindful moments will help you see patterns and progress over time.

4.2 MINDFULNESS MEDITATION: TECHNIQUES AND PRACTICES

Mindfulness meditation comes in various forms, each offering unique benefits. Focused attention meditation involves directing your attention to a single focus point, such as your breath, a word, or an object. The aim is to maintain this focus and gently bring your mind back whenever it wanders. This type of meditation is excellent for improving concentration and reducing mental clutter.

Another form is open monitoring meditation, in which you observe your thoughts, feelings, and sensations without attachment or judgment. This method helps you develop non-reactive awareness, which makes it easier to let go of negative thoughts and emotions.

Loving-kindness meditation (metta) cultivates compassion for yourself and others. You begin with kind thoughts toward yourself and then extend them to loved ones, acquaintances, and even challenging individuals. This practice can significantly boost your sense of empathy and emotional resilience.

Body scan meditation is another effective technique. It involves mentally scanning your body from head to toe, noticing any areas of tension or discomfort. This practice enhances body awareness and promotes relaxation, making it a valuable tool for managing stress and chronic pain.

Let's try out these meditations.

First, set up a comfortable space. Find a quiet spot where you won't be disturbed. You can sit on a cushion or chair or lie down if that's more comfortable.

Keep your back straight but relaxed, and place your hands on your lap or knees.

For focused attention meditation, close your eyes and focus on your breath. Inhale deeply through your nose, and exhale slowly through your mouth. Whenever your mind wanders, gently bring your focus back to your breath.

For open monitoring meditation, sit comfortably and close your eyes. Notice any thoughts or feelings that arise without trying to change them. Observe and let them pass.

In loving-kindness meditation, begin by sitting comfortably and closing your eyes. Take a few deep breaths to center yourself. Start by silently repeating phrases like, "May I be happy, may I be healthy, may I be safe, may I live with ease." After a few minutes, direct these phrases toward someone you love, then to a neutral person, and finally to someone you find difficult.

For body scan meditation, lie down in a comfortable position. Close your eyes and take a few deep breaths. Start by focusing on your toes and noticing any sensations. Gradually move your attention up through your body, spending a few moments on each part. If you notice any tension, imagine breathing into that area and releasing it with each exhale.

Beginners often face challenges like restlessness and distractions. It's normal for your mind to wander, especially when new to meditation. The goal isn't to stop your thoughts but to gently return your attention to the present moment each time your mind drifts. Be patient with yourself. If you find it challenging to sit still—start with shorter sessions, gradually increasing the time as you become more comfortable. Understand that mindfulness is a *practice,* not a quick fix. It takes time to see significant changes. Consistency is more important than perfection.

Finding time for regular practice can be challenging, but even a few minutes a day can make a difference.

Start with short sessions if you have a busy schedule. Even five minutes of focused attention meditation can help you reset and recharge. Use meditation apps and resources for guided sessions and tips. Apps like Calm or Headspace offer various meditations to fit into your day. Combining meditation with other activities can also be effective. Practice mindful breathing while waiting in line, or do a quick body scan before bed. The goal is to make mindfulness a regular part of your routine, helping you stay grounded and present amidst the chaos of daily life.

As you design your 28-day plan, consider including one or more of these meditation practices. A few minutes of body scan meditation or loving-kindness meditation can lay a foundation for emotional balance.

4.3 BODY SCAN MEDITATION FOR ENHANCED AWARENESS

Body scan meditation is a mindfulness practice that helps you tune into your physical sensations by mentally scanning your body from head to toe. Imagine lying comfortably and slowly focusing on each part of your body, noticing any sensations, tensions, or discomforts. This practice aims to bring awareness to areas holding stress or tension, allowing you to release it and promote relaxation. The purpose of body scan meditation is to enhance body awareness and mindfulness, helping you connect more deeply with your physical self. It's like taking an internal tour, offering a moment to check in with your body and understand its needs.

Close your eyes and take a few deep breaths, allowing your body to relax. Begin by focusing on your toes. Notice any sensations you experience. It may be warmth, coolness, tingling, or numbness. Slowly move your attention up to your feet, ankles, and legs. As you scan your body, there's no need to judge or change what you notice. Simply observe with curiosity, breathing gently into any areas of tension and releasing it with each exhale.

Continue this process, moving through your hips, abdomen, chest, arms, hands, neck, and head. Once you've scanned your entire body, take a few deep breaths and slowly open your eyes, bringing your awareness back to your surroundings.

One of the most significant benefits of body scan meditation is enhanced body awareness. Regularly checking in with your body makes you more attuned to its signals and needs. This heightened awareness can help you address physical issues before they escalate. Another benefit is the reduction of bodily tension and pain. By noticing areas of tension and consciously releasing them, you can alleviate chronic pain and discomfort. This practice also promotes relaxation and stress relief. Taking the time to focus on your body and breathe deeply can activate the parasympathetic nervous system, helping you feel calmer and more centered.

There are various ways to practice body scan meditation, allowing you to tailor it to your needs and schedule. For a quick relaxation session, try a short body scan. Spend just a few minutes focusing on the primary areas of your body, such as your feet, legs, abdomen, chest, and head. This scan can be a great way to take a mental break during a busy day.

If you want a more profound experience, an extended body scan might be more suitable. This practice involves spending more time on each body part, allowing for a more thorough exploration and release of tension. You can set aside 20 minutes for this practice, making it a part of your evening routine to help you unwind.

Body scan meditation can also be particularly effective when practiced before sleep. Incorporating a body scan into your bedtime routine can help if you struggle with falling or staying asleep. As you lie in bed, close your eyes and mentally scan your body, releasing all tension. This process can help quiet your mind and relax your body, making it easier to drift off to sleep.

You can also combine body scan meditation with other relaxation techniques, such as progressive muscle relaxation or deep breathing, for an even more effective pre-sleep routine.

Exercise: Quick Body Scan for Stress Relief

Find a quiet space where you won't be disturbed. Sit or lie down in a comfortable position and close your eyes. Take a few deep breaths, allowing your body to relax. Begin by focusing on your toes. Notice any sensations. Gradually move your attention up through your feet, legs, abdomen, chest, arms, hands, neck, and head. Spend a few moments on each body part, observing any tension and imagining it melting away with each exhale.

Once you've scanned your entire body, take a few more deep breaths and slowly open your eyes, bringing your awareness back to your surroundings.

Body scan meditation offers a simple yet powerful way to connect with your body and promote relaxation. A short session for a quick mental break or an extended practice for more in-depth awareness can help you manage stress.

In Week 1 of your 28-day program, body scan meditation is a great tool to cultivate body awareness. You can also use it in Week 4 to reflect on progress and release lingering tension.

4.4 DEVELOPING EMOTIONAL RESILIENCE THROUGH MINDFULNESS

Emotional resilience is your ability to bounce back from stress and adversity. Think of it as your emotional immune system. Just like your physical body fights off illnesses, emotional resilience helps you recover from challenges and setbacks. It's crucial for overall mental health because it enables you to handle life's ups and downs without getting overwhelmed.

Emotional resilience is like a tree bending in the wind—it doesn't resist the storm but flexes with it, returning to its natural state when the winds pass. When emotionally resilient, you can cope with difficulties, adapt to change, and maintain a positive outlook even in tough times. Although resilience may not come naturally, you can cultivate it, and mindfulness is a powerful tool to help you do so.

Mindfulness builds emotional resilience by helping you manage difficult emotions and develop a positive attitude toward challenges. One way it does this is by teaching you to observe your emotions without judgment. When you practice mindfulness, you learn to notice your feelings as they arise without labeling them as good or bad. This impartial awareness enables you to recognize your emotions without becoming entangled.

For example, if you feel anxious, instead of thinking, "I shouldn't feel this way," you might say, "I'm noticing anxiety right now." A shift in perspective can make a huge difference in handling stress.

Developing a mindful attitude towards challenges is another way mindfulness builds resilience. Mindfulness encourages curiosity instead of fear in the face of stress. Challenges become opportunities to learn and grow, not obstacles to avoid. Adopting this mindset allows you to navigate difficulties with greater ease and flexibility. For instance, if you face a setback at work, instead of feeling defeated, you might ask yourself, "What can I learn from this experience?" This approach helps you stay resilient and open to possibilities, even in the face of adversity.

Practical exercises can further enhance your emotional resilience. Mindful breathing is a simple yet effective practice for regulating your emotions. Find a quiet space and sit comfortably. Close your eyes and take a deep breath through your nose, then exhale slowly through your mouth. Focus on the sensation of your breath as it enters and leaves your body. If your mind wanders, gently bring your attention back to your breath.

Mindful journaling is also effective for processing emotions and building resilience. Journaling is like looking in a mirror—only this surface reflects your *inner* world, revealing emotions and patterns that might otherwise go unnoticed.

Set aside a few minutes daily to write about your experiences and feelings. Focus on what you noticed during your mindfulness practice, any challenges you faced, and how you responded to them. This process helps you gain insights into your emotional patterns and develop strategies for managing stress. By reflecting on your experiences, you can identify areas of growth and celebrate your progress.

Mindfulness offers more than just relief from stress—it builds emotional resilience, helping you weather life's storms with greater ease. With every breath and every moment of awareness, you strengthen the foundation for a more balanced and fulfilling life.

The practices shared in this chapter are tools to help you stay grounded, even when life feels chaotic. Building emotional resilience is an ongoing process throughout your 28-day program. Use these mindfulness techniques regularly, especially during moments of stress, to foster resilience and maintain balance.

Reflection Prompt: Mindfulness Techniques and Emotional Resilience

Take a moment to reflect on how mindfulness can enhance your emotional resilience. Use the following questions to guide your journaling or personal reflection:

- Which mindfulness practices introduced in this chapter resonate with you the most? How can you incorporate them into your daily routine?
- Can you recall a recent challenge where mindfulness helped you respond differently? How could you apply these techniques next time?
- What does emotional resilience mean to you, and how can mindfulness support your journey toward building it?

Use these reflections to monitor how mindfulness strengthens your emotional resilience during the 28-day program. Review these notes throughout the program to recognize growth and adjust your practices as needed.

5

SELF-COMPASSION AND SELF-REGULATION

One evening, after the kids were in bed, I was overwhelmed by a wave of self-criticism. My youngest had thrown a tantrum that seemed to last forever, and despite my best efforts—singing, distracting, offering comfort—nothing worked. *Why can't I handle this better?* I thought.

In that moment of despair, I remembered something a fellow mom had once told me: "Treat yourself as you would treat a friend." I paused, took a deep breath, and imagined what I would say to a friend in my shoes. "It's okay," I whispered to myself, "You're doing your best, and it's normal to struggle sometimes." That small act of kindness towards myself was a turning point. It was a powerful reminder of the importance of self-compassion in healing.

From that night on, I made a conscious effort to speak to myself with the same patience and understanding I offered my children. I invite you to consider a moment when you can extend the same kindness to yourself that you so readily offer to others.

5.1 THE ROLE OF SELF-COMPASSION IN HEALING

Self-compassion is a concept developed by Dr. Kristin Neff more than 20 years ago and includes three main components: self-kindness, common humanity, and mindfulness. Self-kindness involves being gentle and understanding with yourself, especially during times of failure or suffering. Instead of harsh self-criticism, you offer yourself warmth and care. Imagine having a bad day, and instead of criticizing yourself, you say, "It's okay to have bad days. You're only human."

Recognizing shared human experience is another crucial aspect of self-compassion. It involves acknowledging that challenges and imperfections are part of the human condition. Understanding that everyone faces difficulties makes being kind to yourself more accessible. This perspective helps you see that you are not alone in your struggles.

Mindfulness, the third component, means being aware of your emotions without judgment—observing your thoughts and feelings as they arise without suppressing or denying them. This nonjudgmental awareness allows you to face your emotions with acceptance and understanding. Imagine noticing a wave of sadness. Instead of pushing it away, you acknowledge it gently, "I see you, and it's okay to feel this way."

Self-compassion is crucial in the healing process for several reasons:

1. It reduces self-criticism and enhances self-worth. When you treat yourself with kindness, you break the cycle of negative self-talk, which can be incredibly damaging. This shift in perspective boosts your self-esteem and self-worth.
2. Self-compassion promotes emotional resilience and stability. By being kind to yourself, you build a stronger emotional foundation, making it easier to navigate life's challenges.
3. Self-compassion facilitates recovery from trauma and stress.

When you approach your pain with compassion, you create a safe space for healing. It's like offering yourself a warm, comforting hug in times of distress.

Scientific evidence supports the benefits of self-compassion. Studies have indicated that self-compassion can reduce anxiety and depression. For instance, a systematic review published in *The Benefits of Self-Compassion in Mental Health* found that self-compassion training significantly improved mental health outcomes, including reduced stress and burnout.

Additionally, research indicates that self-compassion can improve physical health. A study conducted by Dr. Kristin Neff revealed that individuals who practice self-compassion tend to have lower levels of stress and inflammation, promoting better overall health. Furthermore, evidence suggests that self-compassion aids in trauma recovery. By fostering a self-compassionate mindset, individuals can process and heal from traumatic experiences more effectively.

Adopting a self-compassionate mindset involves shifting your perspective from self-judgment to self-kindness. Noticing when you're overly critical of yourself and intentionally responding with kindness and compassion in challenging situations can make a significant difference.

For example, if you make a mistake at work, instead of harshly berating yourself, acknowledge the effort you put in and remind yourself that everyone makes mistakes.

Exercise: The Self-Compassionate Mindset

Next time you catch yourself being self-critical, pause and ask, "How would I speak to a friend in this situation?" Then, offer yourself the same kindness and understanding. Write down a few kind phrases you can use when you need a boost of self-compassion. Keep this list handy and refer to it whenever you need a reminder to be kind to yourself.

Self-compassion is a powerful tool for healing and growth. Treating yourself with kindness, recognizing the shared human experience, and practicing mindfulness can enhance emotional resilience, reduce stress, and support holistic health. Adopting a self-compassionate mindset fosters a deeper connection with yourself.

Incorporate self-compassion exercises during Week 2 of your 28-day program as you focus on emotional regulation. These practices will enhance your ability to stay kind to yourself while navigating emotional highs and lows.

5.2 SELF-COMPASSION EXERCISES: JOURNALING AND REFLECTION

Journaling can be a powerful tool for cultivating self-compassion. It offers a safe space for self-expression, helping you explore your thoughts without judgment. Putting pen to paper creates a private sanctuary for honest reflection. Writing down your experiences lets you process emotions and gain insights into your inner world. By regularly journaling, you develop a habit of reflecting on your day, which can lead to profound self-awareness. Moreover, journaling can be incredibly therapeutic. It allows you to release pent-up emotions and offers relief and clarity.

To get started, consider using specific journaling prompts to encourage self-compassionate writing. One effective prompt is to "Write a letter to yourself from the perspective of a compassionate friend." Imagine a dear friend who knows you well and loves you unconditionally. What would they say to you in a moment of struggle? Write down their words of comfort and encouragement.

Another prompt is to "Reflect on a difficult experience and identify ways you showed resilience." This exercise helps you recognize your strengths and how you've coped with challenges. Lastly, try "List three things you appreciate about yourself today." This simple act of acknowledging your positive qualities can boost your self-esteem and foster a sense of gratitude towards yourself.

Setting up a quiet and comfortable space for journaling is the first step. Find a spot where you won't be disturbed. It could be a cozy corner in your home or a favorite park bench. Make sure you feel relaxed and at ease.

Next, use the prompts to guide your reflections. Start with the one that resonates with you the most. Don't worry about grammar or spelling; just let your thoughts flow freely. After you've written, take a moment to review and revisit your entries.

This practice can help you notice patterns and track your emotional growth over time. Regularly reflecting on your journal entries can deepen your self-compassion and provide valuable insights into your healing process.

In addition to journaling, other reflection techniques can help cultivate self-compassion. Guided self-compassion meditations are a great option. These meditations often involve visualizing a compassionate figure who offers you love and kindness. By regularly practicing these meditations, you can internalize these feelings and develop a more compassionate attitude towards yourself.

Visualization exercises for self-kindness can also be beneficial. Imagine yourself in a peaceful place where you feel completely safe and loved. Visualize yourself receiving kindness and care, and let these feelings wash over you.

Another powerful tool is a daily gratitude practice. At the end of each day, take a few moments to reflect on what you're grateful for, such as a kind word from a friend or a beautiful sunset. Write down three things you're thankful for and notice how this practice shifts your perspective. Focusing on gratitude can help you appreciate the positive aspects of your life and develop a more compassionate outlook towards yourself and others.

Journaling Prompt: Evening Reflection

Each evening, take a moment to reflect on your day. Use this prompt to guide your journaling: *'What were the three most positive moments today? How did I feel during those moments, and what did I learn?'"* This reflection helps you focus on the positive aspects of your day and develop a more self-compassionate mindset.

Use these journaling prompts throughout your 28-day program as part of your evening routine.

In Week 4, revisit earlier reflections to track how your self-compassion has evolved, identifying areas of growth. By incorporating these journaling and reflection techniques into your daily routine, you can develop a more profound sense of self-compassion.

These practices offer a space for self-expression, facilitate self-reflection, and help you process your emotions. Whether it's through writing a letter to yourself, guided meditations, or daily gratitude practice, these exercises will enhance your emotional resilience.

5.3 TECHNIQUES FOR SELF-REGULATION: MANAGING TRIGGERS AND EMOTIONAL STATES

Self-regulation is managing your emotions, thoughts, and behaviors in different situations. Think of it as maintaining emotional balance and stability, which helps you adapt and respond to life's challenges without being overwhelmed. This skill enhances resilience and adaptability, making it easier to bounce back from setbacks.

When you can regulate your emotions, you reduce the impact of stress and trauma on your daily life. Imagine being in a stressful situation, and instead of reacting impulsively, you take a moment to breathe and respond thoughtfully.

The first step in self-regulation is identifying emotional triggers—situations, people, or memories that evoke strong emotional responses. Keeping a trigger journal can be incredibly helpful in this process. When you notice a strong emotional reaction, jot down what happened, how you felt, and any physical sensations you experienced. This practice helps you become more aware of your triggers over time. Keeping a trigger journal throughout your 28-day program will increase your awareness of these patterns over time.

Developing awareness of physical and emotional cues is also crucial. Pay attention to changes in your body, like a racing heart or tight muscles; and your emotions, like sudden anger or sadness. These signals may indicate that you are experiencing a trigger.

Once you've identified your triggers, the next step is to create an action plan for managing them. Start by listing your common triggers and their physical or emotional cues. Then, outline specific strategies to cope with each trigger. For instance, if a particular situation at work triggers anxiety, plan to take a short walk or practice deep breathing when it happens. Having a plan in place can make it easier to manage your reactions and stay in control.

Several self-regulation exercises can help you manage your emotions effectively. Breathwork is a powerful tool for calming the nervous system. One simple technique is the 4-7-8 breathing method. Inhale through your nose for a count of four, hold for a count of seven, and exhale through your mouth for a count of eight. This practice can quickly reduce stress and promote a sense of calm.

Progressive muscle relaxation is another effective exercise. To practice progressive muscle relaxation, start by tensing each muscle group for five seconds, then release. Move from your toes to your head, focusing on the sensation of relaxation spreading through your body. This technique helps release physical tension and promotes relaxation.

Grounding exercises are also valuable for staying present and reducing anxiety. One effective method is the 5-4-3-2-1 technique. Focus on five things you can see, four things you can touch, three things you can hear, two things you can smell, and one thing you can taste. This exercise helps anchor you in the present moment, making it easier to manage overwhelming emotions.

Mindfulness plays a significant role in self-regulation. Practicing mindful awareness of your emotions means observing your feelings without judgment. When you notice a strong emotion, take a moment to acknowledge it without trying to change it. This awareness allows you to respond, rather than react to your triggers.

For example, if you feel anger rising, instead of snapping at someone, you might take a deep breath and calmly express your feelings. Using mindfulness to respond thoughtfully can prevent impulsive reactions and help you maintain emotional balance.

Incorporating mindfulness into your daily routines can enhance your self-regulation skills. Start your day with a few minutes of mindful breathing or a short meditation. Throughout the day, take mindful breaks to check in with yourself. Notice how you're feeling and any physical sensations you're experiencing. This practice helps you stay connected to your body and emotions, making it easier to manage stress and triggers.

In the evening, reflect on your day and any emotional challenges you faced. Consider how you responded and what you might do differently next time.

Mindfulness and self-regulation are deeply interconnected. By practicing mindfulness, you increase your awareness of your emotions and develop the ability to manage them effectively. This combination of awareness and regulation helps you navigate life's challenges with greater ease and resilience.

During the 28-day program, make self-regulation exercises part of your daily routine. Grounding techniques are especially useful in Week 1 for building emotional awareness and stability.

Breathwork, grounding exercises, and daily mindfulness practices can enhance your ability to cope with stress and triggers. Self-regulation is like tuning a guitar—when you're in tune, life's music sounds sweeter, and it's easier to play through the obstacles.

5.4 INTEGRATING SELF-COMPASSION INTO DAILY LIFE

Integrating self-compassion into your daily life can significantly enhance your overall well-being. Imagine starting each day with a supportive inner dialogue instead of a critical one. When you treat yourself with kindness, you reduce stress and promote relaxation.

It's like having a friend who always has your back, no matter what. This consistent support makes handling life's ups and downs easier, helping you build emotional resilience.

Setting Daily Self-Compassion Intentions

Begin your day with a self-compassion intention. It could be as simple as:

- *"I will be kind to myself today."*
- *"I will forgive myself for any mistakes."*

During your 28-day journey, set a self-compassion intention each morning. Use these small rituals to build resilience and develop a habit of treating yourself kindly. This small act sets a positive tone for your day and reminds you to be gentle with yourself. When challenges arise, take a breath and remind yourself:

It's okay to struggle. I deserve kindness.

Celebrate Small Wins

Celebrate even the smallest victories, no matter how minor they seem. Did you manage to complete a task despite feeling anxious? Acknowledge it. Give yourself credit for the effort you put in—it all counts toward your progress.

Creating Self-Compassionate Routines and Rituals

Routines that promote self-kindness can reinforce this habit. Try starting your morning with affirmations like:

- *"I am worthy of love and respect."*
- *"I am doing my best."*

In the evening, take a moment to reflect on your self-compassionate actions that day. Did you take a break when needed? Did you speak kindly to yourself? Acknowledge these moments—they are signs of growth. Incorporating self-care activities, such as taking a warm bath, reading, or making time for a favorite hobby will greatly enhance emotional well-being.

Small Acts that Build Self-Compassion Over Time

Remember, self-compassion isn't about perfection—it's about showing up for yourself, even when things feel hard. Each act of kindness, no matter how small, strengthens your emotional resilience and helps you thrive.

Integrating self-compassion is like planting seeds of kindness in your mind. With time and care, these seeds grow into habits of resilience and self-worth. Every small act of kindness toward yourself is a step toward a stronger, more compassionate you.

Now, let's take a look at Week 2 of your 28-Day Plan.

Instructions for Week 2 Daily Tracker

Welcome to Week 2: Emotional Regulation Through Movement and Breathwork!

This week, we focus on regulating emotions through breathwork and movement. These practices will help you reduce anxiety, relieve stress, and deepen your mind-body connection. Remember that each practice is adaptable—feel free to exchange any exercise for one that better suits your needs. Refer back to Chapter 2 for additional options.

Most importantly, practicing self-compassion as you engage in these exercises is essential for your overall healing.

How to Use Your Week 2 Tracker:

- **Daily Practice Focus**: Each day has a specific focus— breathwork or movement. Review the description of each practice and consider how it meets your needs. Feel free to adapt or exchange exercises as needed.
- **Physical Sensations & Emotional State:** Track physical sensations you notice during each practice. Reflect on your emotional state before and after—how did the practice affect you?
- **Challenges or Insights:** Record challenges you faced or insights you gained. Reflect on your observations—did you feel calmer, more energized, or more connected to your body?
- **Daily Goal/Intention**: Set a goal or intention for each day (e.g., "stay present during yoga" or "practice patience with myself"). This helps keep you focused and engaged.

Daily Practices for Week 2:

- **Day 1:** 4-7-8 Breathing Technique for Anxiety Relief: Inhale for 4 counts, hold for 7, exhale for 8. This helps activate the relaxation response. Feel free to use box breathing or alternate nostril breathing if you prefer.
- **Day 2:** Diaphragmatic Breathing for Relaxation: Place one hand on your belly, inhale deeply, and exhale slowly. This stimulates the vagus nerve, promoting relaxation. If needed, try alternate nostril breathing.
- **Day 3:** Yoga for Emotional and Physical Healing: Try Child's Pose, Warrior II, or Legs-Up-The-Wall. If these poses don't make a difference to how you are feeling, refer to Chapter 2 for other options like Cat-Cow or Savasana.
- **Day 4**: Box Breathing for Stress Reduction: Inhale for 4 counts, hold for 4, exhale for 4, and pause for 4. Repeat to regulate breath and reduce stress. Feel free to substitute with diaphragmatic breathing or 4-7-8 breathing.
- **Day 5:** Tai Chi for Stress Reduction and Body Awareness: Try movements like Wave Hands Like Clouds or Parting the Horse's Mane. Notice how the flow helps you stay present and reduce stress. Switch to other Tai Chi movements if needed.
- **Day 6:** Pilates for Strengthening the Mind-Body Connection: Try The Hundred, or Spine Stretch Forward. Focus on small, precise movements to feel more grounded. If preferred, substitute with other Pilates or gentle yoga stretches.
- **Day 7**: Explore a New Yoga, Pilates, or Tai Chi Movement: Choose a different movement—try Cat-Cow for yoga, Grasp the Bird's Tail for Tai Chi, or Single-Leg Circles for Pilates.

Reflect on how trying something new impacts your connection to your body.

Week 2 Daily Tracker: Emotional Regulation

Day	Practice Focus	Physical Sensations	Emotional State	Challenges/ Insights	Daily Goal/ Intention
1	Breathwork Techniques (e.g., 4-7-8 Breathing)				
2	Diaphragmatic Breathing for Relaxation				
3	Yoga for Emotional and Physical Healing				
4	Box Breathing for Stress Reduction				
5	Tai Chi for Stress Reduction and Body Awareness				
6	Pilates for Strengthening the Mind-Body Connection				
7	Explore a Different Yoga, Pilates, or Tai Chi Movement				

Spreading the Power of Somatic Therapy

"The body is our greatest ally in the healing process, as it holds the wisdom and resources necessary for healing."

— PETER LEVINE

When I discovered somatic therapy, I had heard about the mind-body connection, yet I hadn't really absorbed the information or considered how it could help me. I think there are a lot of things like this… the gut-brain connection, for example. How many times have you heard about this yet let it wash over you without really registering it? The mind-body connection was exactly like that for me. I hadn't experienced it myself, so it was background information, but when I started using somatic therapy, I truly understood its power. I had lived with anxiety for such a long time and tried so many different treatments that I'd begun to believe that nothing would ever work. Somatic therapy showed me just how wrong I was, and I feel so much better now.

The better I felt, the more I realized that I had to help other people to address their trauma with somatic therapy. I'm certainly not saying that other forms of therapy have no value, but for many people, they only address the surface of the issue, and we're sold so many medications that really only treat the symptoms and not the cause. When I discovered just how powerful somatic therapy is, I knew I had to share my knowledge to help other people, and I hope you'll find this as transformative as I have.

Now that we're far enough through our journey together that you can see the potential for healing, I'd like to ask for your help in reaching more people with this information. You can make a huge difference very easily—all you have to do is leave your feedback online.

By leaving a review of this book on Amazon, you'll help new readers who are looking for a realistic and effective way to manage their trauma and pain to find this information and discover the power of somatic therapy.

Not only do reviews help people to find the guidance they're looking for; they tell them about other people's experiences and show them how they could benefit too. So many people are suffering, trying solution after solution to no avail. I believe that somatic therapy can make a real difference, and if we work together, we can help more people find it.

Thank you so much for your support. Your words have power, and I'm so grateful to you for using them for such a good cause.

Scan the QR code below

6

REAL-TIME BIOFEEDBACK AND TECH-BASED TOOLS

I magine sitting at home after a long day, weighed down by stress and anxiety. You've tried deep breathing, meditation, and even a walk, but nothing brings the relief you need. Now, picture having a tool that reveals your body's stress response in real-time—and guides you back to a state of calmness. Heart Rate Variability Biofeedback (HRVB) is a powerful tool that can revolutionize how you manage stress and emotions.

6.1 UNDERSTANDING HEART RATE VARIABILITY BIOFEEDBACK (HRVB)

Heart Rate Variability (HRV) measures the time between heartbeats and reflects your nervous system's balance. Higher variability signals relaxation, while lower variability indicates stress. Heart Rate Variability Biofeedback (HRVB) leverages this by providing real-time data to enhance your emotional and physical health, offering insights into the balance between your sympathetic ("fight or flight") and parasympathetic ("rest and digest") nervous systems.

Practicing HRVB encourages your body to favor a state of relaxation, diminishing the overall impact of stress. HRVB significantly benefits autonomic homeostasis, aiding in maintaining a balanced state that alleviates the symptoms of anxiety and depression and improves the body's response to physical exertion and overall health.

Research, including studies in "Traumatology" and by the National Center for Biotechnology Information (NCBI), confirms HRVB's effectiveness in reducing stress, anxiety, depression, and symptoms of conditions like asthma and irritable bowel syndrome (IBS). It works by optimizing respiratory sinus arrhythmia (RSA) through controlled breathing at a resonance frequency, usually around six breaths per minute, which enhances baroreflex sensitivity and stimulates the vagus nerve, promoting relaxation.

The availability of user-friendly HRVB tools—from wearable monitors like the Polar H10 Heart Rate Sensor, to smartphone apps like HeartMath Inner Balance, and integrated devices like the Apple Watch—has made practicing HRVB very accessible. These tools provide real-time HRV feedback and come with various features, including guided meditations and in-depth data analysis, appealing to those seeking a comprehensive view of their autonomic function.

HRVB presents a scientifically supported method for effectively managing stress and emotional health. With such a wide range of accessible tools, from wearables to apps and desktop devices, HRVB empowers individuals to enhance their heart rate variability for better stress management and emotional regulation.

For beginners, start with a device like the Polar H10 chest strap or the Apple Watch. These tools are easy to use and provide reliable feedback on your HRV. The accompanying apps will guide you step-by-step in interpreting your results.

HRVB is incorporated into Week 3 of the 28-day program. Real-time feedback will help you stay attuned to your body's responses and adjust your techniques to promote relaxation.

6.2 USING HRVB FOR STRESS MANAGEMENT AND EMOTIONAL REGULATION

Imagine unwrapping a new HRVB device—its sleek design promises a new path toward managing stress and regulating emotions. The first step is simple: secure the device comfortably on your body, be it a chest strap, ear sensor, or wristband. Then, sit quietly to let it record your baseline heart rate variability (HRV)—the crucial starting point for your journey.

Interpreting HRVB data might initially appear complex, but accompanying apps simplify this process, guiding you through metrics like heartbeat intervals and overall HRV scores—key indicators of your autonomic nervous system's balance.

These apps provide personalized feedback, set goals, and suggest breathing exercises tailored to your stress levels and emotions. The most impactful HRVB exercises involve synchronized breathing guided by your device's feedback. Inhaling and exhaling slowly, about five seconds, aligns your breathing with the device's rhythm to enhance HRV and shift towards relaxation. Incorporating visualization—imagining serene scenes like a tranquil beach or a quiet forest—can further deepen your calm state.

Another effective technique is progressive relaxation, where you tense and then relax different muscle groups in sequence, from toes to head, while observing your HRV responses. This not only aids physical relaxation but also cultivates a deeper understanding of how bodily tension influences HRV, ultimately improving your emotional self-regulation.

Consistent HRVB practice promises significant benefits, including sustained stress reduction, bolstered emotional resilience, and heightened self-awareness. Through regular use, you train your body to manage stress better, leading to a more balanced autonomic nervous system and informed decision-making around stress and emotional management.

During the 28-day program, incorporate HRVB exercises at the start and end of your day to enhance emotional awareness and balance. Record your baseline HRV and monitor improvements throughout the program.

Integrating HRVB into your routine involves a blend of correct setup, targeted exercises, and consistent practice. By accurately measuring your baseline, engaging in exercises like synchronized breathing and progressive relaxation, and regularly reviewing your progress, you leverage HRVB for long-term stress alleviation, emotional resilience, and enhanced self-awareness.

This approach, supported by real-life examples and scientific research, positions HRVB as an invaluable asset in navigating tension and cultivating emotional balance. HRVB is like learning to ride a bike —once you get the rhythm, it becomes second nature, helping you steer through stress with greater ease.

6.3 MINDFULNESS APPS: CHOOSING AND USING THE BEST TOOLS

Consider those days when nothing seems to go right. Work was a grind, personal commitments piled up, and now you just want to unwind.

Mindfulness apps offer a solution. These digital tools provide guided meditations, breathing exercises, and sleep aids. Mindfulness apps bring the benefits of mindfulness right to your fingertips, making it accessible anytime, anywhere. They are your pocket-sized meditation coach, ready to guide you through a quick meditation session or remind you to take a mindful breath.

Mindfulness apps can help you manage stress, improve focus, and promote better sleep. Popular mindfulness apps like Calm, Headspace, Insight Timer, and MyLife offer a range of features to support your mindfulness practice.

Calm, for example, is well-known for its soothing sounds of nature and guided sleep stories, perfect for winding down after a long day. Calm offers new meditations, moves, and breathing exercises daily. Headspace provides a structured approach to mindfulness, with courses designed to build your skills over time. Insight Timer boasts a large library of free content, including guided meditations from teachers worldwide. MyLife (formerly Stop, Breathe & Think) offers personalized mindfulness plans based on your current mood and needs.

Using these apps can transform your mindfulness practice. The guided meditations make starting easy, even if you're new to mindfulness. The tracking features allow you to monitor your progress, giving you a sense of accomplishment. Reminders help you build a consistent practice, ensuring that mindfulness becomes a regular part of your routine. Plus, the variety of content available means you can always find something that resonates with you, whether it's a quick 60-second breathing exercise or a longer meditation session.

When choosing a mindfulness app, several criteria can help you find the best fit for your needs. First, consider the user interface and design. A user-friendly app with an intuitive layout makes it easier to navigate and use regularly. Look for apps that offer a range of features, such as guided meditations, progress tracking, and reminders. Customization options are also important, allowing you to tailor the content to your preferences and goals. Finally, reviews and user feedback can provide valuable insights into the app's effectiveness and reliability. Apps with high ratings and positive reviews are generally a safer bet.

There are many fantastic mindfulness apps. Calm is my go-to app because it offers everything I need in one place. Calm offers guided meditations, sleep stories, soothing soundscapes, and videos on relaxing stretches and mindful movement. Its clean, user-friendly design makes it easy to navigate, and I appreciate being able to track my progress. The app also sends gentle reminders and check-ins throughout the day, helping me stay mindful of my emotions and consistent with my practice.

Headspace offers a more structured approach, with courses designed to build mindfulness skills progressively. It also includes features like "SOS" meditations for moments of panic or stress. Insight Timer is ideal for those who want a wide variety of content. With thousands of guided meditations from different teachers, you can find something that suits your mood and needs.

MyLife stands out for its personalized approach. The app asks you to check in with your emotions and offers tailored mindfulness plans based on your responses.

If you're unsure which app to choose, consider starting with a free trial or exploring Insight Timer's free offerings. Each app has unique strengths—Calm focuses on sleep and relaxation, and Headspace offers a structured course.

Integrating mindfulness apps into your daily routine can be a game-changer. Start by setting daily reminders for your mindfulness practice. Most apps allow you to schedule notifications, gently prompting you to be mindful. Combining app-based practices with other somatic exercises can enhance the benefits. For instance, you might use a guided meditation from Calm after a yoga session or practice a breathing exercise from Headspace before starting your day.

Using apps during short breaks and downtime can also be effective. Instead of scrolling through social media, take a few minutes to practice mindfulness, allowing you to reset and recharge.

Many apps offer features that allow you to monitor your meditation streaks, track your moods, and see your overall progress. Use this data to reflect on what works best for you and adjust as needed. If you notice that specific meditations are more effective, focus on those. If practicing at a particular time of day yields better results, adjust your schedule accordingly.

Experiment with short mindfulness sessions during daily activities. For example, use a breathing exercise from your app during lunch breaks or listen to a guided meditation while commuting.

Whether you're looking to reduce stress, improve focus, or simply take a mindful moment, these apps offer a convenient and accessible way to support holistic health.

6.4 INTEGRATING BIOFEEDBACK AND APPS INTO YOUR HEALING ROUTINE

Imagine concluding a long, stressful day with work, errands, and personal commitments. Combining biofeedback and mindfulness apps helps manage stress by enhancing self-awareness and promoting consistent practice. Biofeedback devices offer real-time insights into your HRV, showing how stress affects your body. Mindfulness apps complement this by guiding you through meditations and breathing exercises.

To reap the full benefits, integrate regular HRVB sessions into your week, aiming for three to four times, and embed mindfulness exercises into your daily routine for a balanced approach. Addressing both physiological and psychological stress allows for adjustments based on real-time feedback. For instance, if certain practices improve your HRV, include more of them in your routine.

Tracking your HRV scores, feelings, and observations before and after each session helps refine your approach. Combining biofeedback with mindfulness apps creates a holistic strategy for stress management and emotional regulation. This practice deepens your understanding of your physical and emotional states, empowering you to make well-informed decisions about your well-being.

During Week 3 of the 28-day program, explore different mindfulness apps to enhance your experience. Guided meditations can complement your biofeedback sessions, helping deepen emotional awareness and build resilience. Use this time to experiment with tech-based tools, reflecting weekly on how HRVB and mindfulness apps impact your progress. Adjust as needed to ensure these practices align with your goals and support your growth.

With these tools, you're ready to face whatever challenges come your way. Every mindful breath and heartbeat will strengthen your emotional resilience, building a sustainable practice that supports you through life's ups and downs.

Reflection Prompt: Real-Time Biofeedback and Tech-Based Tools

As you think about the tools and strategies introduced in this chapter, take a moment to reflect on how they might enhance your healing journey. Use the following questions to guide your journaling:

- How comfortable do you feel integrating tech-based tools like HRVB or mindfulness apps into your routine?
- What practices—such as biofeedback or guided meditation—resonate most with you? How can you incorporate them into your daily life?
- In what ways can real-time feedback support your emotional regulation or stress management goals?

This reflection will help you assess how to use biofeedback and mindfulness apps effectively, empowering you to create a balanced, tech-enhanced healing routine.

7

ADVANCED SOMATIC PRACTICES

Picture this: you're standing in the middle of a bustling city, surrounded by the sounds of construction, hurried footsteps, and distant chatter. The chaos makes your heart race, your breath quicken, and your body tense. Now, imagine stepping into a quiet park nearby, finding a peaceful spot beneath a tree, and focusing on your breath. Slowly, your heartbeat steadies, your breath deepens, and the tension in your muscles begins to melt away. The power of advanced breathwork techniques can guide you from the edge of overwhelm to a place of profound peace and emotional release.

7.1 ADVANCED BREATHWORK TECHNIQUES FOR DEEP HEALING

Unlike simple breath awareness or basic techniques like box breathing, advanced breathwork involves complex patterns and requires a more substantial commitment. These techniques can bring significant emotional release, physical detoxification, and spiritual insights. Advanced breathwork techniques are like the deep ocean—mysterious, powerful, and capable of unlocking hidden emotional treasures.

For those ready to explore these depths, advanced breathwork offers a transformative experience.

One such technique is Holotropic Breathwork, developed by Dr. Stanislav Grof. This method involves continuous, deep, and rapid breathing, often accompanied by evocative music. The goal is to reach an altered state of consciousness where deep emotional and physical healing can occur.

During a Holotropic Breathwork session, you lie down comfortably and begin by taking deep breaths quickly. The facilitator guides you, ensuring you maintain the rhythm and depth of your breath. As the session progresses, you may experience intense emotions, vivid memories, or physical sensations. This technique can lead to profound emotional release and a sense of catharsis.

It's crucial, however, to have a trained facilitator present to guide and support you throughout the process.

Rebirthing Breathwork is another advanced technique that focuses on addressing birth-related trauma. Developed by Leonard Orr, this method involves circular breathing, with no pause between the inhale and exhale. The continuous flow of breath helps release suppressed emotions and trauma from early life experiences. During a session, you lie down and breathe in a connected, circular pattern. The facilitator may guide you through visualizations or prompts to help you access and release birth-related memories.

Shamanic Breathwork offers a distinctive approach for those seeking spiritual healing. It combines deep breathing with shamanic drumming and guided imagery. The practice connects you with inner wisdom and facilitates spiritual insights. During a session, the rhythm of your breath aligns with the drumming, guiding you through visual journeys. These journeys may bring encounters with spirit guides or reveal transformative insights, fostering emotional release and deeper spiritual connection.

Transformational Breathwork, developed by Dr. Judith Kravitz, focuses on creating cognitive shifts and enhancing overall well-being. This technique involves conscious, connected breathing, where the inhale is active and the exhale is passive. The goal is to clear blockages in the body and mind, allowing for greater clarity and transformation. During a session, you lie down and breathe in a connected pattern, focusing on the sensations in your body. The facilitator may use affirmations, movement, or acupressure to enhance the experience. Transformational Breathwork can lead to cognitive shifts, increased self-awareness, and a sense of empowerment.

While advanced breathwork techniques offer profound benefits, they also have potential risks. The intense emotional release and physical sensations can be overwhelming for some individuals. Hyperventilation is a common risk, leading to dizziness, tingling, or even loss of consciousness if not managed properly. Therefore, it's essential to approach these techniques with caution and under the guidance of a qualified breathwork facilitator.

Finding a trained and experienced facilitator is crucial for ensuring a safe and supportive environment. They can guide you through the process, help you navigate intense emotions, and provide grounding techniques if needed.

Creating a safe and comfortable environment for your breathwork practice is also necessary. Choose a quiet, private space where you won't be disturbed. Use comfortable cushions or blankets to support your body, and have water and tissues nearby. Recognize and respect your limits. If you feel overwhelmed or uncomfortable at any point, it's okay to take a break or stop the session.

Always listen to your body and honor its signals.

Post-session care is equally important. After a breathwork session, you may feel emotionally raw or physically tired. Taking time to ground yourself is essential. Grounding techniques like walking barefoot on grass, drinking water, or eating a nourishing meal can help bring you back to the present moment. Journaling about your experience can provide insights and help integrate the emotional release. Self-care practices like taking a warm bath, resting, or engaging in gentle movement can support your body and mind as you process the session.

Whether you're exploring Holotropic Breathwork, Rebirthing Breathwork, Shamanic Breathwork, or Transformational Breathwork, these practices can lead to profound insights and transformation. Approaching these techniques with caution, under the guidance of a qualified facilitator, and focusing on self-care can ensure a safe and supportive experience.

For those who prefer to practice without a facilitator, there are advanced yet simplified breathwork techniques you can safely explore independently. Conscious Connected Breathing involves continuous, deep breaths without pauses between inhaling and exhaling. This technique allows you to access deeper emotional layers by creating a rhythmic energy flow through your body. Practice lying down in a comfortable space, focusing on maintaining an even, unbroken breath pattern for several minutes at a time.

Cyclic Sighing is another powerful technique combining a long, deep inhale through your nose and an extended sighing exhale through your mouth. This helps release built-up tension and access deeper relaxation.

Although these practices can be done individually, they induce strong emotional and physical responses. Take your time and allow yourself to ease into these techniques gradually.

Always listen to your body and practice post-session care.

7.2 SOMATIC EXPERIENCING: RELEASING TRAUMA THROUGH BODY AWARENESS

Somatic Experiencing (SE) offers a profound way to address trauma stored in the body. Imagine the tightness in your chest or lump in your throat—these sensations often carry unresolved emotional weight. Unlike traditional "talk therapy", SE taps into the body's innate ability to heal by renegotiating trauma through bodily awareness and gentle interventions.

The foundational concept is that trauma isn't just a mental or emotional experience; it lives in the body, manifesting as physical sensations, tension, and discomfort. By addressing these bodily experiences, SE aims to release stored trauma and restore balance.

In a typical SE session, the process begins with tracking bodily sensations. You might start by sitting or lying down in a comfortable position. The therapist encourages you to observe physical sensations like warmth, tingling, or tightness. Developing this awareness is essential for recognizing how your body stores trauma.

Next comes "pendulation," the gentle movement between feelings of comfort and discomfort. This technique helps you build tolerance for distressing sensations without becoming overwhelmed. For instance, if you feel tightness in your chest, the therapist might guide you to shift your focus to a more neutral or pleasant sensation, like the warmth in your hands. This back-and-forth movement helps regulate your nervous system and gradually releases stored tension. If you're practicing pendulation alone, try identifying a point of discomfort and then intentionally shifting your focus to a neutral or comforting area of your body. Gently move your attention between these sensations, taking breaks if necessary, and remain compassionate with yourself throughout the process.

"Titration" is another crucial technique in SE, involving the gradual release of trauma in small, manageable doses. Imagine emptying a full bathtub by letting out just a trickle of water at a time. This slow process prevents you from becoming overwhelmed by intense emotions or sensations. During a session, the therapist might ask you to focus on a mildly distressing memory or sensation, guiding you to stay with it briefly before shifting your focus to something neutral or positive. This controlled exposure helps your nervous system process and release trauma without triggering a full-blown stress response.

"Resourcing" is an essential component of SE, providing you with internal and external tools to create a sense of safety and stability. Resources such as a comforting memory, a favorite place, or a supportive person can make you feel calm and secure. During a session, the therapist might guide you to visualize your resources, helping you anchor your body and mind in a safe, grounded state and building your capacity to handle distress.

You can try practical SE exercises at home to enhance your body awareness and release tension patterns. Start with a grounding exercise through sensory awareness. Sit comfortably and focus on your breath. Notice the sensation of your feet on the ground, the weight of your body on the chair, and the feeling of your clothes against your skin. This simple exercise helps anchor you in the present moment, reducing anxiety and promoting relaxation.

Introduce SE practices in Week 3 of your 28-Day Program when exploring more advanced techniques. Try grounding exercises or pendulation to regulate your nervous system after emotionally intense days.

Another exercise involves identifying and releasing tension patterns. Lie down and perform a body scan, starting from your toes and moving up to your head. Notice tension or discomfort, and imagine breathing into those areas, releasing the tension with each exhale. This practice helps you become more aware of how your body holds on to stress and provides a pathway for releasing it.

Imagery exercises can also support safe trauma processing. Close your eyes and visualize a place where you feel completely safe and relaxed. It could be a beach, a forest, or a cozy room. Notice the details of this place—the colors, sounds, and sensations. Spend a few minutes immersing yourself in this safe space, allowing your body to relax and your mind to feel calm. Visualizations serve as a resource during challenging moments, helping you stay grounded and centered.

Somatic Experiencing offers significant benefits, especially for those dealing with PTSD and complex trauma. Research shows that SE can effectively reduce symptoms of PTSD, depression, and anxiety by addressing the physical manifestations of trauma. It helps restore the body's natural ability to self-regulate, promoting a sense of safety. However, SE does have its limitations. While it excels in addressing the physical and emotional aspects of trauma, it may not fully address the cognitive components, such as negative thought patterns or beliefs.

Additionally, SE is most effective when guided by a professional, especially for those with severe trauma. Self-guided practices can be beneficial, but the presence of a trained therapist ensures safety and provides more in-depth insights into the healing process.

Incorporating Somatic Experiencing into your healing journey can offer profound relief from trauma stored in the body. You can gradually release tension and restore balance by tracking bodily sensations, using techniques like pendulation and titration, and building resources. Practical exercises such as grounding through sensory awareness, identifying and releasing tension patterns, and using imagery for safe trauma processing can enhance your body awareness and support your healing process.

While SE has limitations, its focus on the body's innate ability to heal makes it a powerful tool for those seeking to overcome trauma and build a stronger mind-body connection.

7.3 EMBODIMENT PRACTICES: FULLY INHABITING YOUR BODY

Imagine walking through life feeling fully present. Every step, every breath, every sensation can be experienced with complete awareness. This is the essence of embodiment. In somatic therapy, embodiment means being fully present and aware of your body. It's about feeling every sensation, understanding how your emotions manifest physically, and connecting deeply with yourself.

Being fully present allows you to tune into the subtle signals your body sends, helping you better navigate emotions and stress.

Embodiment practices enhance this connection between physical sensations and emotions. Like learning a new dance, the steps might initially feel unfamiliar, but over time, you move with grace, fully present in each moment.

One powerful technique is Authentic Movement. This practice involves moving spontaneously without any predefined steps or choreography. You close your eyes and let your body guide you, moving however it wants to. The idea is to listen to and express your body's impulses through movement. Often, this is done with a witness who holds space and observes without judgment. This witnessing can be incredibly validating, helping you feel seen and understood.

Authentic Movement allows you to explore and express emotions that might be difficult to articulate with words.

Bonnie Bainbridge Cohen developed Body-Mind Centering, another approach to embodiment. This practice integrates awareness of body systems, such as the skeletal, muscular, and organ systems. Focusing on how these systems feel and move helps you better understand your body's internal landscape. For example, you might explore the sensation of your bones supporting your body, or the rhythm of your breath moving through your lungs.

Integrated awareness helps you connect with your body on multiple levels.

Continuum Movement, founded by Emilie Conrad, emphasizes fluidity and connection. This practice involves slow, wave-like movements that mimic natural patterns found in water and other elements. The goal is to dissolve rigid patterns in the body and mind, allowing for greater flexibility and ease. You might start by lying on the floor and gently swaying your body, feeling the fluid motion ripple through you. Continuum Movement encourages you to feel the interconnectedness of your body, enhancing your sense of flow and connection.

Contact Improvisation takes embodiment to a relational level. This dance form involves two or more people moving together, exploring physical contact and shared movement. It's a dance of listening and responding, where you continuously adapt to your partner's movements. This practice enhances your awareness of others and builds trust and communication. For instance, you might start by leaning into your partner, feeling their support, and offering your own. As you move together, you develop a deep connection and relational awareness.

Embodiment practices have profound benefits. They enhance body-mind integration, helping you understand how physical sensations and emotions are intertwined. This integration promotes emotional expression and release, allowing you to process and let go of stored emotions. By tuning into your body, you build resilience and adaptability.

Let's look at some practical exercises to help you explore embodiment.

Find a quiet space for an Authentic Movement session and close your eyes. Begin by tuning into your breath and noticing any sensations in your body. When you feel ready, start moving in whatever way feels natural. Let your body guide you without any judgment or expectation. If possible, have a witness present to observe your movement.

After the session, take a few moments to reflect on your experience, either through journaling or discussing it with your witness.

For readers new to these techniques, try a simplified version of Authentic Movement: Set a timer for five minutes and move your body freely to soothing music, without judgment.

In Body-Mind Centering, you can try an exploratory exercise focusing on your skeletal system. Lie down and close your eyes. Bring awareness to your bones, starting with your feet and moving up through your body. Notice the sensation of your bones supporting you. Feel the structure and stability they provide. Connecting with the foundational aspects of your body promotes a sense of groundedness and support.

For Continuum Movement, start with a fluid movement sequence. Sit or lie down in a comfortable position. Begin by gently swaying your body like a wave moving through water. Allow this movement to ripple through your entire body, feeling the fluid connection between different parts. Tune into the sensations and let the movement flow naturally. This practice helps dissolve rigid patterns and promotes fluidity and relaxation.

Contact Improvisation can be explored with a partner. Start by standing or sitting close to your partner and gently lean into each other. Feel the support and connection between you. Begin to move together, responding to each other's movements. Let the dance evolve naturally, without any predefined steps. Contact Improvisation enhances your awareness of others and builds a deep sense of trust and connection.

Embodiment practices offer a powerful way to fully inhabit your body and connect with your emotions. Integrating techniques like Authentic Movement, Body-Mind Centering, Continuum Movement, and Contact Improvisation enhances body-mind integration, promotes emotional expression, and builds resilience.

Incorporate a brief Authentic Movement or Body-Mind Centering session during Week 3 of your 28-Day Program. Journaling after these sessions can enhance your insights.

These practices deepen your relationship with your body.

Polyvagal Theory builds on this foundation, illuminating the intricate dance between emotional regulation and the nervous system's responses to stress.

7.4 EXPLORING POLYVAGAL THEORY IN SOMATIC THERAPY

Developed by Dr. Stephen Porges, Polyvagal Theory offers a fascinating lens through which to understand emotional regulation and how our bodies respond to stress. At its core, this theory revolves around the vagus nerve—a crucial component of the parasympathetic nervous system. The vagus nerve plays a significant role in controlling the heart, lungs, and digestive tract, but it's also intricately linked to our emotional responses. Polyvagal Theory breaks down the autonomic nervous system into ventral vagal, sympathetic, and dorsal vagal. Each state has its own set of characteristics and responses to stress, which can profoundly influence how we feel and behave.

The ventral vagal state is where we ideally want to be most of the time. It's associated with feelings of safety, social engagement, and relaxation. When you're in this state, you're calm, connected, and able to engage with others effectively. Imagine sitting with a close friend, feeling relaxed and at ease—that's your ventral vagal system at work.

Conversely, the sympathetic state is the "fight or flight" mode, which kicks in when you perceive a threat, real or imagined. Your heart rate speeds up, your muscles tense, and you're ready to act. Think of the adrenaline rush you feel when narrowly avoiding a car accident.

Lastly, the dorsal vagal state is often called the "shutdown" mode. This state occurs when stress is so overwhelming that one feels immobilized or disconnected. Some experience this as being frozen in fear.

Polyvagal Theory is incredibly relevant to somatic therapy because it provides a framework for understanding how our nervous system responds to stress and trauma. Techniques stimulating the ventral vagal state can help you feel safer and more connected. Recognizing signs of sympathetic arousal, such as increased heart rate or sweating, can alert you when you're in fight or flight mode.

Similarly, noticing signs of dorsal shutdown, like feeling numb or disconnected, can help you understand when you're in a freeze state. By identifying these states, you can use specific strategies to move between them safely and effectively.

Let's discuss some Polyvagal-informed exercises you can try. Vagal breathing involves slow, deep breaths that stimulate the vagus nerve and promote relaxation. Sit comfortably and inhale deeply through your nose for a count of four. Hold your breath for a count of four, then exhale slowly through your mouth for a count of six. Repeat this cycle several times, and you'll likely feel calm and centered.

Another powerful tool is the Safe and Sound Protocol (SSP), an auditory intervention developed by Dr. Porges. This involves listening to specially filtered music which stimulates the vagus nerve and enhances emotional regulation. The music is designed to promote feelings of safety and calm, making it easier to engage socially and manage stress.

Co-regulation practices can also be incredibly beneficial. These involve engaging in calming activities with a partner or therapist. For example, you might sit back-to-back with a partner and synchronize your breathing. Feeling their breath rise and fall in tandem with yours can create a sense of connection and safety.

Enhancing self-regulation is one of the most significant advantages of using Polyvagal Theory. By understanding how your nervous system responds to stress, you can use specific techniques to bring yourself back to a state of balance. However, there are challenges, too.

Understanding and applying the theory can be complex, especially without guidance. The nuances of recognizing different states and knowing how to respond can be tricky. For those dealing with severe trauma, professional guidance is crucial. A trained therapist can help you navigate these states safely and provide insights into your healing process.

Polyvagal Theory offers a roadmap to emotional regulation through the lens of the nervous system. By recognizing signs of sympathetic arousal, dorsal shutdown, or ventral vagal calm, you gain insight into your emotional states. Tools like vagal breathing, co-regulation, and the Safe and Sound Protocol empower you to respond intentionally to stress. Although applying the theory can be complex, its benefits make it a valuable resource for deep healing.

These advanced somatic practices—breathwork, Somatic Experiencing, embodiment techniques, and Polyvagal Theory—offer profound ways to reconnect with your body and heal deeply. With practice and guidance, you can move through emotional challenges, foster resilience, and unlock new levels of emotional freedom. The tools are here; your healing journey awaits.

Reflection Prompt: Advanced Somatic Practices

As you reflect on the advanced somatic practices shared in this chapter, take a moment to consider the following questions:

- Which advanced practice—such as Holotropic Breathwork, Somatic Experiencing, or Polyvagal Theory—resonates most with you, and why?

- How can you incorporate elements from these techniques into your existing healing routines?
- What emotions, sensations, or insights arise when you imagine trying one of these practices? How might they enhance your emotional resilience or deepen your self-awareness?

Instructions for Week 3: Advanced Somatic Practices, Biofeedback, and Tech-Based Tools

Welcome to Week 3 of your 28-Day Program! This week, you'll explore advanced somatic practices and integrate real-time biofeedback and mindfulness apps into your routine.

How to Use Your Week 3 Tracker

- **Daily Practice Focus**: Each day focuses on a specific practice to explore advanced somatic techniques, embodiment practices, or tech-based tools. Adapt or exchange practices based on what feels best for you. Refer to Chapters 6 and 7 for more options. Consider incorporating a challenging movement sequence, such as advanced yoga or Pilates.
- **Physical Sensations & Emotional State**: Track physical sensations and emotions during each practice. Note changes in heart rate, tension, or relaxation. Did using biofeedback or advanced breathwork bring more clarity or calm?
- **Challenges or Insights**: Record any challenges or insights. Was it difficult to sync with the biofeedback device? Did a practice help you connect with your emotions?
- **Daily Goal/Intention**: Set a daily goal, like "improve HRV through deep breathing" or "focus on releasing tension during SE exercises."

Daily Practices for Week 3

- **Day 1: Advanced Breathwork** (e.g., Holotropic or Transformational Breathwork, or Cyclic Sighing): Use deep, rhythmic breathing to reach deeper relaxation and emotional release. If this feels intense, refer to Chapter 2 for simpler breathwork.

- **Day 2: Somatic Experiencing (Body Awareness and Pendulation)**: Practice pendulation by moving between sensations of discomfort and comfort to build emotional resilience. Notice how this affects your emotional state.

- **Day 3: Embodiment Practice** (e.g., Authentic or Continuum Movement): Engage in an embodiment practice to explore and express bodily sensations. Move freely without predefined steps. If too challenging, revisit gentle stretching or yoga from earlier weeks.

- **Day 4: Self-Compassion Practice (Journaling, Reflection, or Visualization)**: Spend time cultivating self-compassion and explore ways to ensure you will use it daily. For a quick reminder on self-compassion exercises, refer to Chapter 5.

- **Day 5: Polyvagal Theory (Vagal Breathing & Co-Regulation)**: Use slow, deep breaths to stimulate the vagus nerve, and practice co-regulation with a partner to enhance connection. Notice the impact on emotional regulation.

- **Day 6: Heart Rate Variability Biofeedback (HRVB)**. Use a biofeedback tool like the Apple Watch or Polar H10. Record your baseline HRV and practice resonance breathing. Observe how your breathing affects your HRV and relaxation. Try your favorite exercise with HRVB.

- **Day 7: Integrating HRVB with Guided Meditation**: Explore different mindfulness apps. The guided meditations complement biofeedback sessions by deepening emotional awareness. Combine HRVB with a guided meditation from an app like Calm or Headspace. Reflect on how real-time feedback affects your presence and relaxation.

Week 3 Daily Tracker: Advanced Somatic Practices, HRVB, and Tech-Based Tools

Day	Practice Focus	Physical Sensations	Emotional State	Challenges/ Insights	Daily Goal/ Intention
1	Advanced Breathwork (e.g., Transformational Breathwork or Cyclic Sighing)				
2	Somatic Experiencing (Body Awareness and Pendulation)				
3	Embodiment Practice (e.g., Authentic or Continuum Movement)				
4	Self-Compassion Practice (Journaling, Reflection, or Visualization)				
5	Polyvagal Theory (Vagal Breathing & Co-Regulation)				
6	Heart Rate Variability Biofeedback (HRVB)				
7	Integrating HRVB with Guided Meditation (Mindfulness Apps)				

8

INTEGRATING SOMATIC PRACTICES INTO DAILY LIFE

Have you ever walked into a room and felt a sense of calm? It could be a cozy living room bathed in warm light or a minimalist bedroom where everything was perfectly in place. That sensation isn't just a coincidence—your environment profoundly influences your emotions. Creating a somatic-friendly environment at home can enhance your healing journey by making it easier to engage in calming and restorative practices.

8.1 CREATING A SOMATIC-FRIENDLY ENVIRONMENT AT HOME

Your home can serve as a sanctuary where you leave daily stresses behind and connect with yourself through somatic practices. A well-organized, intentional space promotes relaxation, making it easier to focus on healing. Clutter, on the other hand, can create mental noise, subtly raising stress levels. Reducing clutter isn't just about tidiness— it helps clear your mind, preparing you for deeper engagement with your practices. Whether it's a corner in your living room, or an entire room dedicated to your sessions, having a designated space mentally primes you to move into your practice quickly.

Incorporate elements that promote relaxation to enhance the comfort and effectiveness of your space. Calming colors like soft blues, greens, or lavender soothe the mind. Choose natural light or soft, warm lighting. Comfortable furniture that supports your body is essential—whether it's a yoga mat, meditation cushion, or a favorite chair. Plants like lavender, aloe vera, or snake plants improve air quality and infuse the space with a sense of peace and connection to nature.

Sensory enhancements can elevate the atmosphere further. Aromatherapy, for example, offers a subtle yet powerful way to shift your emotional state. Essential oils like lavender, chamomile, or eucalyptus can create an environment of tranquility. Use a diffuser, or place a few drops on a cotton ball to enjoy the calming aroma. Sound also plays a role—gentle rain, ocean waves, or soothing piano melodies. Apps like *Calm* offer soundscapes and background music to enhance your practice.

Textures also matter. Soft blankets, cozy rugs, and comfortable clothing can make your space more nurturing. Think about how comforting it feels to wrap yourself in a blanket at the end of a long day—bringing that sense of physical ease into your somatic space encourages more profound relaxation.

Maintaining this environment is as important as creating it. Regular decluttering and seasonal adjustments keep the space fresh and relevant to your needs. In the summer, switch out heavy blankets for lighter ones; add cozy touches like candles or throws in winter. Keeping your space well-maintained ensures it remains a personal, supportive refuge.

Even though decluttering can feel daunting—especially during stressful moments—it can immediately be calming. Even when I'm exhausted or reluctant, cleaning my space always leaves me feeling lighter and more at ease. A maintenance routine makes this easier to manage: a quick daily tidy-up, a deeper weekly clean, or a monthly refresh keeps your environment inviting and stress-free.

Checklist: Setting Up Your Somatic Space

- Declutter: Remove items that don't serve a purpose.
- Calming Colors: Use soothing colors like blue, green, or lavender.
- Natural Light: Arrange your space near a window, if possible.
- Comfortable Furniture: Invest in a quality yoga mat, meditation cushion, or cozy chair.
- Natural Elements: Add a variety of plants.
- Aromatherapy: Use essential oils such as lavender or chamomile.
- Soft Sounds: Play background music or nature sounds that resonate with you.
- Textures: Incorporate soft blankets, rugs, and comfortable clothing.
- Regular Maintenance: Schedule weekly tidying and seasonal updates.

Following this checklist will ensure your home becomes a supportive space for your life and practices.

8.2 DAILY RITUALS FOR CONTINUOUS HEALING AND GROWTH

Rituals act as anchors in your day, creating a sense of consistency and grounding. They structure tasks and your emotional well-being, helping you stay connected and mindful. Rather than merely checking off items on a to-do list, these small, intentional practices cultivate stability and comfort.

Over time, even seemingly minor rituals—like a morning stretch or an evening reflection—can build meaningful change and support personal growth.

Morning Rituals: Starting the Day with Intention

How you begin your day sets the tone for everything that follows. A morning ritual doesn't need to be elaborate—simple practices can help ease you into your day with presence and clarity.

Start with gentle stretches to wake up your body. Take a moment to stretch your arms, legs, and back before leaving bed. A quick stretch loosens any stiffness from sleep and signals to your mind and body that the day is beginning.

Following your stretch with breathwork or meditation can deepen your sense of calm. Sit comfortably, close your eyes, and take a few slow breaths. Focus on the sensation of your breath moving in and out, letting any tension melt away with each exhale. Even just five minutes of mindful breathing can create a foundation of clarity and focus.

Setting daily intentions brings purpose to your actions. Take a moment to reflect on what you hope to accomplish—in terms of tasks and how you want to feel and engage with the day. Ask yourself: *What energy do I want to carry with me? What do I hope to experience today?* This small act can shift your mindset, making the day more intentional and meaningful.

Evening Rituals: Unwinding and Reflecting

Just as a morning routine sets the tone for the day, evening rituals provide an opportunity to wind down and release stress. After a busy day, your body and mind need time to transition to rest. An evening body scan is a simple way to relax. Lie down in a quiet space and slowly move your attention through your body, starting at your toes and moving up to your head. Breathe into any areas of tension, allowing the stress to soften with each exhale.

Reflective journaling at the end of the day can also be therapeutic. Use this time to write about what went well, any challenges you encountered, and how you felt throughout the day. This process helps you process emotions and provides insights into patterns and growth.

Calming activities like sipping herbal tea or a warm bath can further enhance your evening routine. These simple acts signal to your body that it's time to relax. A warm bath soothes tense muscles, while a cup of chamomile tea promotes restful sleep.

Transition Rituals: Shifting with Purpose

Transition rituals are small but impactful practices that help you smoothly shift between different parts of your day. These moments of intentional transition prevent stress from spilling over from one activity to the next, helping you stay present. For example, a short meditation after work can help you leave professional stress behind and fully re-engage with your personal life. Take a few minutes to sit quietly, close your eyes, and breathe deeply. As you exhale, visualize yourself releasing any lingering work-related thoughts. Gratitude practices at meal times can also foster mindfulness. Before eating, pause to reflect on what you are grateful for. Whether it's the food in front of you, the company you're with, or the simple joy of resting, this moment of appreciation helps cultivate a positive mindset.

Mindful walking is a very effective transition practice. Instead of rushing through your break, take a slow, intentional walk. Pay attention to each step, the sensations in your body, and the environment around you. This simple act grounds you in the present moment.

Building a Sustainable Ritual Practice

Daily rituals needn't be complicated to be effective. The key is consistency—small, repeated practices create meaningful change over time. Start by identifying the rituals that resonate with you. Choose natural and supportive practices, such as morning meditation, mindful walks, or journaling at night.

Rituals offer more than just structure—they are acts of self-compassion. Morning rituals gently awaken your body and mind, while evening routines allow you to reflect, release, and reset. These small moments of intention build a foundation for healing.

Integrating these rituals into your routine offers moments of reflection and connection, helping you stay grounded even during life's busiest moments. As you develop these habits, you'll notice subtle shifts in your emotional well-being and a deeper connection with yourself.

Focus on creating morning and evening rituals that support emotional regulation and reflection. Use breathwork or body scans during these rituals to connect with your emotions. Track how these rituals enhance your well-being in your journal.

What is one small ritual you could begin tomorrow? How might this ritual support your healing goals? Write down your thoughts and commit to trying it for the next three days.

With consistent practice, daily rituals become second nature. The benefits will soon become apparent as these practices anchor you in the present and support your ongoing personal development.

8.3 MINDFUL MOVEMENT IN EVERYDAY ACTIVITIES

Mindful movement involves staying present and fully engaged in physical activities, turning everyday moments into opportunities for greater awareness. Rather than prioritizing speed or intensity, it encourages you to focus on each motion—how it feels and how your body responds.

This intentional approach helps build body awareness, enhances coordination, and reduces stress by allowing you to tune into your body's needs. When practiced consistently, mindful movement transforms ordinary actions into moments of connection, fostering a sense of ease and balance throughout your day.

Incorporating Mindful Movement into Daily Life

Incorporating mindful movement doesn't require drastic changes to your routine. Everyday activities—when done with intention—become opportunities to stay grounded.

Remember mindful walking? Instead of rushing from task to task, slow down and pay attention to each step. Feel the ground beneath your feet, notice the movement of your muscles, and sync your breath with your pace. Even a short walk to the mailbox can become a grounding exercise when you stay present.

You can also practice mindfulness while doing household chores. Focus on your breath while washing dishes, vacuuming, or folding laundry. Inhale deeply through your nose and exhale slowly through your mouth, allowing these repetitive tasks to become moments of calm and reflection. These small shifts make mundane chores feel more purposeful and will help reduce stress.

Gentle stretching throughout the day is another way to engage with mindful movement. Whether sitting at a desk or taking a break, stretch your arms, legs, and back. Pay attention to how your muscles feel as they move, using each stretch as a chance to reset and refresh.

Activities That Naturally Encourage Mindful Movement

Some activities lend themselves naturally to mindful movement, such as dancing. Dance is a joyful way to connect with your body and emotions. Put on your favorite song and let your body move freely. Notice how the rhythm influences your movements and how your body responds. Dancing with loved ones can make this practice more enjoyable and spontaneous.

One of my favorite things to do is dance with my kids. We play silly music and let loose, moving however we like. It's a beautiful way to connect, share laughter, and fill the house with joy.

Staying Present Through Mindful Movement

Here are a few simple strategies to help you stay connected to your body throughout the day:

- **Body Check-Ins**: Set reminders on your phone to pause and notice how you feel. Are your muscles tense or relaxed? Do you need a moment to stretch or breathe deeply? These check-ins help you stay aware of your body's signals.
- **Mindfulness Prompts**: Place sticky notes with words like "Breathe" or "Relax" in visible places, such as on your computer or bathroom mirror. These reminders encourage brief moments of centering throughout the day.
- **Gratitude for Movement**: Take a moment to appreciate what your body does for you each day—whether walking, dancing, or stretching. Cultivating gratitude for movement deepens your connection to your body and supports emotional well-being.

Small, intentional shifts can have a significant positive impact. Start with micro-practices, such as taking three deep breaths while waiting for your coffee or stretching your neck while seated.

With time and consistency, these practices will become second nature.

8.4 BALANCING WORK, LIFE, AND SOMATIC PRACTICES

Balancing multiple responsibilities can be overwhelming, making it difficult to prioritize self-care. Competing priorities can lead to burnout without intentional stress management, but brief somatic practices throughout the day can help.

Quick desk exercises like seated Cat-Cow stretches or neck rolls can relieve tension, while mindful breathing offers grounding in stressful moments. Use work breaks for gentle movement, such as stretching, or a body scan, to re-energize and boost productivity.

Balancing personal life with somatic practices can be enjoyable when approached creatively. Involving your family in mindful activities turns self-care into shared moments of connection. Invite your family for a short yoga session or a five-minute breathing exercise before bedtime.

A family nature walk provides a fabulous opportunity to practice mindfulness together. Show your family how to focus on the colors, sounds, and smells around you to stay present. Nature has a calming effect, helping to reduce stress and enhance mood. Whether it's a walk in the park, a hike in the woods, or simply sitting under a tree, immersing yourself in a natural environment can help ground you and rejuvenate your mind and body. Embracing nature as part of your self-care routine benefits both your physical and emotional health. Enjoying it with family is like icing on the cake.

Carving out time for yourself is equally important. Whether you take a quiet walk, enjoy a favorite book, or simply sit in silence, these small acts of self-care recharge you for other responsibilities.

Prioritizing your well-being enhances your presence and effectiveness, allowing you to be your best self for both you and your family.

Setting Realistic Goals and Healthy Boundaries

Maintaining balance requires realistic expectations and clear boundaries. Use a planner or digital calendar to schedule time for somatic practices, giving them the same priority as work meetings or family events. Being intentional with your schedule ensures that self-care doesn't get pushed aside.

Saying no to unnecessary commitments is also essential for preserving balance. It's easy to overextend yourself, but learning to decline tasks or invitations that don't align with your priorities prevents burnout. Balancing work, life, and self-care requires flexibility, creativity, and a commitment.

Integrating brief somatic exercises into your workday, involving family in mindful activities, and setting realistic goals are small but meaningful ways to nurture balance.

Each small action—a mindful breath, a stretch, or a walk—adds value. With intention and practice, these moments will accumulate, creating a more manageable and fulfilling life. Take a breath, move mindfully, and trust you're on the right path.

Reflection Prompt: Integrating Somatic Practices into Daily Life

As you reflect on the practices shared in this chapter, consider how you might integrate them into your daily life. Use the following questions to guide your reflection:

- What small changes can you make in your environment to create a more calming and supportive space?
- Which daily rituals—whether in the morning, evening, or between tasks—resonate most with you? How can you begin incorporating them?
- How might mindful movement during everyday activities, such as walking or household chores, enhance your sense of presence?
- What realistic boundaries or adjustments could you set to balance your responsibilities while prioritizing somatic practices?

These reflections will help you identify meaningful ways to weave somatic practices into your routine, making self-care a natural and sustainable part of your life.

9

COMMUNITY AND SUPPORT

Healing doesn't happen in isolation. It thrives within relationships—whether with friends, family, therapists, or even entire communities. As you engage in somatic practices, building connections with others becomes an essential part of your growth.

This chapter explores cultivating a supportive network, leveraging online resources, and discovering the power of sharing your journey with others. With the right people by your side, your healing can become a shared experience enriched by empathy and collective strength.

9.1 THE IMPORTANCE OF CONNECTION IN HEALING

Human beings are wired for connection. Our nervous systems respond to the presence of others, which is why meaningful relationships are so critical in healing. Supportive connections provide comfort, help us process emotions, and offer perspective during tough times. Sharing our struggles and triumphs with others reinforces that we are not alone, easing the burden of healing.

Interpersonal connections play a unique role in somatic therapy. A shared hug, eye contact, or the simple presence of a trusted person activates the ventral vagal system—the part of the nervous system responsible for feelings of safety and social engagement. Spending time with loved ones, participating in support groups, or working with a therapist can accelerate emotional recovery.

However, fostering meaningful connections takes effort. It's not just about having people around—it's about engaging with them intentionally. Sharing thoughts, setting boundaries, and asking for support are essential to maintaining healthy relationships. Healing can feel overwhelming, but knowing someone is walking alongside you makes the process more manageable.

Relationships also offer space for co-regulation—the experience of soothing your nervous system through connection with others. Shared moments, such as sitting quietly with a friend, enjoying a meal with family, or participating in a group session, promote emotional regulation and create a sense of belonging.

Practical Tip: Pay attention to how your body feels when spending time with different people. Do you feel calm, energized, or tense? This awareness can help you identify relationships that nurture your well-being, and those that may need adjustment.

Building meaningful connections doesn't mean having a large or extensive social circle. Quality matters more than quantity. A few trusted people—friends, family, or a therapist—can support you.

Recognize that healing is not a solo endeavor; it's woven through the relationships that offer understanding, presence, and care.

9.2 BUILDING A SUPPORT NETWORK: FRIENDS, FAMILY, AND THERAPISTS

Imagine having a safety net of people who genuinely care about your well-being. A well-rounded support network goes beyond conversations—it's about feeling understood and having others help lighten your load. Friends and family can offer emotional comfort and practical assistance, such as listening, helping with tasks, or simply being present. Having the support of people who care about you can significantly ease the challenges during difficult times.

Therapists provide specialized support, helping you process emotions and develop personalized strategies. A skilled therapist offers more than a sympathetic ear—they create a space where you can explore your experiences without fear of judgment. This professional guidance plays a key role in building emotional resilience and progressing in your healing.

A clear dialogue with your loved ones helps them support you effectively. Communicate your needs and boundaries—whether it's asking for quiet time after therapy or explaining how they can best assist you. Sharing the basics of somatic therapy with them can also foster understanding. Inviting family or friends to join activities such as yoga sessions or mindful walks creates shared experiences that strengthen your relationships and healing.

Choosing the right therapist is essential. Look for someone experienced in somatic therapy and ask key questions during consultations, such as, "How do you adapt techniques for individual clients?" Setting clear goals ensures you and your therapist work toward the same outcomes.

Maintaining a healthy support network requires communication and balance. Regular check-ins with loved ones inform them of your progress and evolving needs. Be mindful of their capacity, too—encourage them to care for themselves and seek support when needed. If your support system feels insufficient, consider expanding it through new therapists, groups, or online communities.

Reflection Section: Assessing Your Support Network

- Who provides emotional or practical support?
- What are your needs, and how can you communicate them?
- How can loved ones participate in activities that aid your healing?
- What criteria will help you choose the right therapist?
- How often will you check in with your network?
- How can you maintain balance and avoid burnout in your relationships?

A well-balanced support network, including friends, family, and therapists, provides the foundation for sustainable healing. You can cultivate relationships that foster growth through clear communication, shared activities, and professional guidance.

9.3 ONLINE COMMUNITIES AND RESOURCES

Online communities provide a valuable way to connect with others who understand your experiences, regardless of location. These platforms offer continuous access to support, whether you're in a rural area or a bustling city. The anonymity of online forums can also make it easier to open up without fear of judgment.

Communities like Reddit's **r/traumatoolbox** and Facebook groups dedicated to somatic healing offer spaces to exchange advice, share stories, and receive encouragement. Specialized forums on platforms like **PsychCentral** provide reliable, moderated environments for discussing trauma and mental health.

While these spaces offer connections and resources, they also come with challenges. Misinformation can spread, and the absence of face-to-face interaction may limit trust. Additionally, excessive screen time can add to stress rather than alleviate it.

To navigate these communities safely:

1. Verify the credibility of the platform.
2. Look for moderation by professionals or clear guidelines for participation.
3. Establish boundaries for your online engagement to prevent overwhelm and protect your privacy by limiting personal information shared publicly.

Online communities complement in-person support by offering diverse perspectives and convenient access. Engaging thoughtfully with these platforms allows you to benefit from shared wisdom while maintaining emotional balance.

9.4 SHARING YOUR JOURNEY: THE POWER OF COLLECTIVE HEALING

There's something incredibly powerful about sharing your own story. When you open up about your experiences, you create a ripple effect, touching the lives of others in ways you might never have imagined. Sharing your personal stories can foster a sense of collective healing. It's like throwing a pebble into a pond; the ripples spread far and wide, creating connections through shared experiences. By telling your story, you can inspire and motivate others. Moreover, sharing helps you gain new perspectives and insights. Hearing how others interpret your experiences or how they relate them to their own lives provides a fresh lens through which to view your own challenges.

Choosing the right platform to share your story is crucial. Depending on your comfort level, you might opt for in-person sharing, online forums, or even written formats like blogs or journals. In-person sharing can be incredibly impactful, offering immediate feedback and emotional connection. Online platforms provide a broader audience and the convenience of sharing from the comfort of your home.

Writing your story can also be therapeutic, allowing you to organize your thoughts and reflect deeply on your experiences. Structuring your narrative for clarity and impact is essential. Start with a clear introduction, share the key events and emotions, and conclude with the lessons learned, or the progress made. Be mindful of your boundaries and privacy. Only share what you're comfortable with, and remember that keeping certain details to yourself is always okay.

The benefits of collective healing are profound. When you share your story, you contribute to a community where empathy and compassion thrive. Hearing others' experiences can strengthen your emotional resilience—just knowing you're part of a supportive network. This shared support encourages continuous personal growth. Every story you hear, and piece of advice you receive adds to your toolbox of coping strategies and insights. This collective wisdom can be incredibly empowering, helping you confidently navigate your own path.

Members often share their journeys in support groups, offering insights and support. One member might talk about how they've used mindfulness techniques to manage anxiety; while another shares their experience with somatic exercises to release stored trauma. These exchanges create a rich tapestry of experiences and strategies, offering a wealth of knowledge and insight to everyone involved. Testimonials from support group members often highlight the sense of belonging and understanding that comes from this kind of sharing.

Sharing your story is a powerful way to foster healing—for yourself and others. Whether in person, online, or through writing, these connections help cultivate resilience and emotional growth. Every shared experience enriches the collective, contributing to a stronger, more compassionate community.

Reflection Prompt: Community and Support

Take a moment to reflect on the connections that support your healing journey. Use the following questions to guide your thoughts:

- Who are the people in your life who provide emotional or practical support? How do these relationships impact your well-being?
- How might you enhance your connections to foster even deeper healing?
- What role could online communities play in expanding your support network?
- If you were to share some of your personal story, what insights or experiences would you feel comfortable offering? How might sharing your journey inspire both yourself and others?

This reflection will help you identify ways to strengthen your relationships, cultivate meaningful connections, and actively participate in a community that nurtures your healing.

- **Body Check-Ins**: Set reminders on your phone to pause and notice how you feel. Are your muscles tense or relaxed? Do you need a moment to stretch or breathe deeply? These check-ins help you stay aware of your body's signals.
- **Mindfulness Prompts**: Place sticky notes with words like "Breathe" or "Relax" in visible places, such as on your computer or bathroom mirror. These reminders encourage brief moments of centering throughout the day.
- **Gratitude for Movement**: Take a moment to appreciate what your body does for you each day—whether walking, dancing, or stretching. Cultivating gratitude for movement deepens your connection to your body and supports emotional well-being.

Instructions for Week 4: Integration and Resilience Building

You've made it to Week 4! This week focuses on integrating what you've learned and building resilience for long-term change. You can integrate somatic habits into your daily routine by developing rituals, practicing mindful movement, and adapting somatic techniques into everyday activities.

How to Use Your Week 4 Tracker

- Daily Practice Focus: Each day focuses on integrating somatic practices into your daily routine. Establish a somatic-friendly environment, establish morning and evening rituals, practice mindful movement, use transition rituals, and reflect on your progress.
- Physical Sensations & Emotional State: Track physical sensations and emotions during and after each practice. Notice how these practices affect you in real-life contexts— are you more at ease during transitions? Are certain rituals helping you feel more grounded?
- Challenges or Insights: Note any challenges or insights as you adopt these practices. If activities are difficult to integrate or rituals are challenging to establish, then reflect on why that might be. Small adjustments, like adding music or taking mindful walks, can make a big difference.
- Daily Goal/Intention: Set a goal or intention for each day, such as "stay present while dancing" or "use a transition ritual to relax after work."

Daily Practices for Week 4

- **Day 1: Create a Somatic-Friendly Environment**—Declutter, add calming elements like soft lighting or aromatherapy, and ensure your space supports your practices.

- **Day 2: Morning Ritual**—Establish a morning ritual, such as gentle stretching or breathwork, to start your day with intention.
- **Day 3: Transition Rituals & Evening Ritual**—Create transition rituals to smoothly transition between activities, such as meditation, to move from work to personal time. Establish an evening ritual like a body scan or reflective journaling to wind down before sleep.
- **Day 4: Mindful Movement in Daily Activities and Chores**—Practice mindful movement during daily activities (walking or dancing) and household chores (emptying the dishwasher or folding clothes) to cultivate mindfulness. Notice your breath and stay fully present.
- **Day 5: Staying Present through Mindful Movement**—Use body check-ins, mindfulness prompts, and gratitude for movement.
- **Day 6: Balancing Responsibilities**—Integrate somatic practices into a busy schedule, like taking short breaks for stretching or involving family in mindful activities.
- **Day 7: Reflection & Resilience Building**—Reflect on your progress throughout the week and the entire program. Consider what has worked well, what you'd like to continue, and how these practices have supported your resilience. Integration is about sustaining these beneficial habits in your daily life.

Week 4 Daily Tracker: Integration and Resilience Building

Day	Practice Focus	Physical Sensations	Emotional State	Challenges/ Insights	Daily Goal/ Intention
1	Creating a Somatic-Friendly Environment				
2	Morning Ritual to Start the Day with Intention				
3	Transition Rituals and Evening Ritual				
4	Mindful Movement—Daily Activities (e.g., Walking, Dancing) and Household Chores				
5	Staying Present through Mindful Movement				
6	Balancing Responsibilities and Integration				
7	Reflection and Resilience Building				

I O

SUCCESS STORIES AND CASE STUDIES

Picture a summer evening, the sky dark and still, as everyone waits for the first burst of fireworks. Each brilliant explosion draws cheers, lighting the night with vibrant colors. Well, this chapter is like that fireworks display—each success story illuminating the transformative power of somatic therapy. This chapter features four categories of success: individuals healing from PTSD, overcoming anxiety, managing chronic pain, and cultivating personal growth through somatic practices.

10.1 TRANSFORMATIONAL STORIES: HEALING FROM PTSD

Ray, a Marine injured by two explosive devices, exemplifies the resilience of the human spirit. After witnessing his best friend's death and suffering from Traumatic Brain Injury (TBI), Ray developed severe PTSD. His struggles with chronic pain, depression, cognitive challenges, and night terrors left him emotionally exhausted. With the guidance of Dr. Peter Levine, Ray began Somatic Experiencing (SE), starting with simple grounding exercises like breath awareness and feeling his feet on the ground. As these practices reduced the intensity of his flashbacks, Ray gradually incorporated body awareness exercises, helping him release trauma stored in his nervous system. Eventually, he became confident enough to participate in a healing retreat for veterans. "Somatic therapy reconnected me with my body and gave me a path to healing," Ray reflects.

Another survivor of multiple traumas found comfort through yoga and mindfulness. Living in a near-constant state of hypervigilance, they struggled with anxiety and intrusive thoughts. Their therapist introduced them to gentle yoga poses like Child's Pose and Legs-Up-the-Wall, which gave them a sense of safety. Mindfulness meditation complemented these practices, helping them observe their thoughts without judgment. "The grounding exercises were a lifeline during panic attacks," they share. Over time, these techniques built emotional stability, helping them reconnect with their body and reduce anxiety.

A first responder, overwhelmed by years of trauma, discovered the restorative power of Tai Chi. Their flashbacks and hyper-alert state gradually softened as they practiced movements like "Wave Hands Like Clouds." Focusing on slow, intentional motion and breath awareness brought physical relaxation and mental calm. "I never thought I could feel this much peace again," they reflect. Through daily practice, Tai Chi became a vital tool for managing PTSD and restoring emotional balance.

These stories highlight the importance of consistency, and trust in the healing process. Grounding exercises like breath awareness anchor individuals in the present moment, reducing flashbacks. Breathwork techniques, such as the 4-7-8 method, provide immediate relief during moments of distress. Tai Chi and yoga promote body awareness, offering physical and emotional release. Developing a routine with these practices will foster resilience and empowers individuals to take control of their healing journey.

10.2 OVERCOMING ANXIETY: REAL-LIFE SUCCESSES

Sarah, a professional juggling a demanding career, struggled with crippling anxiety. Presentations and meetings triggered panic, and social situations left her paralyzed by fear. She found relief through body scan meditations, which helped her identify and release physical tension. "Mindfulness meditation changed my relationship with anxiety," she shares. This practice allowed her to approach professional challenges more calmly and clearly, transforming her work environment into a space she could manage much more confidently.

Michael, a university student, faced overwhelming exam stress that spilled into every part of his life. Simple tasks like attending lectures became a source of dread. Pilates provided the structure he needed to manage his anxiety. Focusing on movements like The Hundred and Roll-Up helped Michael reconnect with his breath, promoting physical and mental stability. "Pilates gave me a sense of control," he reflects, crediting the practice to improving his academic performance *and* emotional well-being.

Emily, a parent navigating the challenges of daily life, found herself debilitated by frequent panic attacks. Grocery shopping and school events felt overwhelming. She turned to the 4-7-8 breathing technique, which quickly became her go-to tool during panic attacks. "Breathwork gave me back control," Emily shares. Over time, the practice reduced both the severity and frequency of her anxiety episodes, empowering her to engage more fully in daily activities.

These stories show how somatic techniques address specific challenges. Mindfulness meditation helped Sarah ease social anxiety; Pilates provided Michael with a sense of structure and control; and breathwork offered Emily immediate relief from panic attacks.

Consistent practice empowered each of them to manage anxiety effectively and build emotional resilience.

10.3 SOOTHE CHRONIC PAIN: CASE STUDIES AND INSIGHTS

Alex, a professional soccer player, faced debilitating chronic pain after a severe hamstring injury sidelined him from the sport he loved. Traditional treatments offered little relief, so he turned to yoga and breathwork. Gentle poses like Downward Dog and Pigeon Pose eased his muscle tension, while diaphragmatic breathing promoted relaxation. "Yoga restored my mobility and reduced my pain," Alex shares. His practice alleviated his pain and also strengthened his mental resilience, allowing him to return to the field with renewed energy.

Laura, an office worker suffering from chronic lower back pain, found that prolonged sitting had taken a toll on her body. She began practicing yoga to stretch her muscles and strengthen her core. Poses like Cat-Cow and Bridge provided much-needed relief. Over time, her pain diminished, and her quality of life improved. "Yoga allowed me to move freely again," Laura reflects, grateful for the return of her physical well-being.

George, a retiree managing arthritis, discovered the benefits of Tai Chi. The gentle, flowing movements improved his joint flexibility and reduced stiffness. "Tai Chi became my lifeline," he shares, finding physical relief *and* emotional support through the community classes he attended. The practice helped him stay active and connected, enhancing his overall outlook and well-being.

These stories emphasize the role of somatic therapy in managing chronic pain. Yoga offers flexibility and strength, Tai Chi promotes joint health and relaxation, and breathwork reduces muscle tension. Each individual found relief through consistent practice, reclaiming their ability to move comfortably and enjoy life again.

10.4 PERSONAL GROWTH AND RESILIENCE THROUGH SOMATIC THERAPY

Lisa, a young adult battling self-doubt, found empowerment through Pilates. Her slumped posture mirrored her lack of confidence, but the focus on breath and movement gradually transformed her mindset. "Pilates made me feel strong and confident in my body," Lisa shares. This newfound strength extended into her daily life, allowing her to engage more assertively at work and in social settings.

David, a high-achieving professional, struggled with burnout and chronic stress. Mindfulness meditation and breathwork became essential tools for managing his emotions. "Mindfulness gave me the tools to handle stress gracefully," he reflects. By observing his thoughts without judgment, and practicing breath control, David cultivated resilience in his professional and personal life.

A senior seeking to reclaim her vitality, Helen turned to Tai Chi and yoga. Gentle movements helped her regain physical strength, while breath-centered practices renewed her emotional well-being. "Somatic practices brought joy back into my life," Helen reflects, embracing her later years with newfound energy and enthusiasm.

These individuals exemplify how somatic practices will foster personal growth. Pilates empowered Lisa to overcome self-doubt, mindfulness gave David the tools to manage stress, and Tai Chi and yoga helped Helen reconnect with her body. Each practice offers more than physical relief—it nurtures emotional resilience and ultimately enriched their lives.

Conclusion

Whether managing PTSD, anxiety, chronic pain, or personal growth challenges, somatic therapy offers tools for transformation. Each individual's journey reflects the power of resilience, showing that it's possible to reclaim well-being and live fully once more with the proper support and dedication.

Reflection Prompt: Success Stories and Case Studies

Take a moment to reflect on how the stories in this chapter resonate with your own personal experiences.

- What somatic practices from these stories inspire you to explore or deepen your practice?
- How do the challenges and successes shared in these case studies relate to your journey?
- What role can resilience and consistency play in your healing process?
- How might sharing your progress or challenges with others—whether through conversations or online support groups—enhance your growth?

Reflections like this will help you identify practices that align with your needs and cultivate resilience. Consider the good value of sharing your healing journey with others.

A Letter to Future You

As we conclude this chapter, I have a small request to make—but first, a bit of background.

At the end of my senior year of high school, my English teacher gave us an assignment: "Write a letter to your future self. In four years, I'll mail it to you. What do you want to tell your future self? Maybe it's what you hope to accomplish, what you're excited or worried about, or what you want to work toward. What advice can you offer? Write about who you are right now—your passions, dreams, and challenges."

It was the most memorable assignment I've ever received—one that left a lasting mark on me. I poured my heart and soul into that letter, unsure what life would look like when I finally read it.

Four years later, while visiting home from college, the letter arrived—addressed to me in my own handwriting. I tore it open with sheer excitement, having forgotten all about it. As I read my words, tears filled my eyes—not tears of sadness, but of hope, joy, and pride. I felt grateful for my progress and at peace with the ongoing process of becoming the person I had always hoped to be.

That letter became a time capsule of who I was, and what I hoped to become, offering renewed insight and perspective. Now, I want to offer you the same gift of reflection and encouragement.

Here is my request:

Take a moment to envision where you want this pursuit of balance to lead. Then, find a pen and write a letter to your future self. Celebrate the progress you hope to make with somatic practices, but also who you are right now. Include the challenges you're navigating, the steps you're taking, and the tools you use. Most of all, offer words of encouragement, the kind that will inspire and uplift you as you continue forward.

When the time feels right, revisit the letter—whether it's a month, a year, or several years from now. Reflect on how far you've come, embrace your progress, and remember to be kind and loving to yourself along the way.

The process of becoming your truest self is unfolding, one step at a time. Your future self will thank you for starting today.

11

MAINTAINING LONG-TERM WELL-BEING

Imagine you're building a house. You've laid a solid foundation, but regular upkeep is essential to keep it standing strong. Just as consistent maintenance preserves a home, continuous practice sustains your progress through therapy, preventing setbacks, and strengthening your ability to handle new challenges. It's important not to wait for distress to return before practicing the somatic techniques that keep you well.

11.1 LONG-TERM STRATEGIES FOR EMOTIONAL AND PHYSICAL HEALTH

Daily self-care is like adding insulation to your house—it sustains your progress and keeps you functioning optimally. Mindfulness practices, like meditation and breathwork, help maintain a calm and centered mind. Movement routines such as yoga, Tai Chi, or a simple walk keep your body strong and your mind clear. Good nutrition and hydration are also key to supporting emotional and physical health.

Regular self-check-ins are like routine house inspections, ensuring everything stays in good condition. Weekly reflections through journaling help you connect with your thoughts and emotions, while monthly reviews provide a broader perspective on your progress. These practices will create a sustainable routine to support your long-term well-being.

Building a lifestyle that supports well-being also means prioritizing rest, meaningful relationships, and joyful pursuits. Restful sleep, uplifting social connections, and engaging in hobbies all contribute to emotional resilience and physical health, creating a balanced life.

11.2 REVISITING AND REVAMPING YOUR HEALING PLAN

As you would know by now, life brings constant change, and your healing plan must evolve with it. Regularly reviewing and updating your plan ensures it aligns with your current needs. Techniques that once helped may no longer serve you, and new challenges may emerge. This process is a bit like tuning a musical instrument—regular adjustments keep everything in harmony.

Set aside time periodically to reflect on your progress and adjust your practices as needed. Be honest about what's working, and perhaps what isn't. Incorporate fresh practices to keep your healing plan engaging—whether it's adding new movement practices or modifying routines to match your current needs. Seeking input from a therapist or support group will offer valuable perspectives and suggestions for improvement.

11.3 CONTINUOUS LEARNING AND GROWTH IN SOMATIC PRACTICES

Continuous learning is essential for maintaining progress and building resilience. Staying informed about new developments in somatic therapy expands your practice and ensures you're using the most effective methods. Books, online courses, and professional conferences will all deepen your understanding and inspire new approaches to somatic techniques.

Engaging with the broader somatic community also fosters growth. Connecting with peers through forums or workshops provides fresh perspectives, support, and motivation. Regularly experimenting with new techniques and reflecting on their impact helps keep your practice dynamic and meaningful.

11.4 STAYING MOTIVATED: TIPS AND TRICKS

Maintaining motivation can be challenging, especially when the demands of 21st century life overwhelm you. Setting short- and long-term goals provides structure and direction. Tracking your progress visually—through a journal or an app—helps keep you motivated when challenges arise.

Celebrate small wins along the way. Treat yourself to something special or take time to reflect on your progress. Inspirational quotes, motivation apps, and support from an accountability partner can also help you stay on track. During any difficult times, focus on small steps rather than pushing yourself too hard, and stay compassionate with yourself—setbacks are part of the process.

11.5 CELEBRATING MILESTONES AND PROGRESS

Celebrating milestones reinforces your motivation and confidence. It's a reminder that your hard work yields results. Whether it's treating yourself to something special, sharing your achievements with loved ones, or reflecting in a journal, acknowledging your ongoing progress keeps you connected to your personal journey.

Tracking your progress visually, whether through a journal or a calendar, also makes your achievements tangible. Marking anniversaries of key accomplishments helps you stay connected to your growth and reinforces your commitment to long-term well-being.

11.6 OVERCOMING SETBACKS AND CHALLENGES

Setbacks are going to be inevitable, but they don't represent failure—instead, they offer opportunities for growth. Reframing setbacks as learning experiences helps you gain clarity on what went wrong and *why*, prompting adjustments that will strengthen your approach.

Seeking support from a therapist, friend, or support group can provide encouragement and insights during difficult times. Simple practices like mindfulness, yoga, or gratitude exercises can help you stay grounded and maintain optimism, turning setbacks into stepping stones for even more joyful and positive future growth.

11.7 THE FUTURE OF SOMATIC THERAPY: TRENDS AND INNOVATIONS

Advances in technology are transforming somatic therapy, making self-care more accessible. Biofeedback tools, AI-powered mindfulness apps, and wearable devices are changing how we monitor and manage stress. These innovations integrate wellness practices seamlessly into daily life.

Holistic approaches that combine somatic therapy with complementary modalities are also gaining prominence, offering more comprehensive care. Staying connected to these trends—through reading, attending events, or engaging with online communities—ensures you remain informed and, more importantly, *inspired* in your practice.

11.8 EMPOWERING YOURSELF FOR A RESILIENT LIFE

Empowerment is key to lasting resilience. Taking charge of your healing builds confidence and a sense of self-efficacy. Setting and achieving personal goals reinforces your progress and strengthens your commitment to well-being.

Practices like affirmations, visualization, and goal-setting exercises help you stay focused and motivated. Self-compassion is also crucial —treat yourself with the kindness you'd offer a friend, especially when facing challenges. These empowerment practices create the foundations of resilience, helping you thrive in the face of inevitable obstacles and maintain long-term well-being.

Final Reflection Prompt: Empowering Your Future Self

Reflect on your journey so far:

- What strengths have you discovered through your healing process?
- What empowering goals will guide you in the months to come?
- How can you show yourself compassion during moments of uncertainty?

Use these reflections as touchstones to stay connected with your growth, trusting that each small step you take will build the resilient, empowered life you envision.

DAILY ROUTINE PLANNER WORKSHEET

This planner is designed to help you create a sustainable daily routine. Use the fillable fields below to integrate somatic practices, mindful activities, and other supportive exercises into your daily life. Adjust these routines as needed to fit your schedule and evolving needs.

Morning Ritual

Daily Intention Setting: *(e.g., Today, I will focus on being present)*

____

Activity: *(e.g., Mindful breathing, stretching, affirmations)*

____

Midday Check-in Activity

Activity: *(e.g., Grounding exercise, HRVB practice)*

____

Self-Compassion Reminder

Reminder: *(e.g., I am doing my best, and that is enough)*

____

Evening Wind-Down Practice

Activity: *(e.g., Body scan, gratitude journaling)*

____

Daily Affirmation

Affirmation: *(e.g., I am worthy of care and healing)*

____

Self-Reflection at Night

Reflection: *(e.g., What made me feel most grounded today?)*

____

Daily Intentions, Affirmations, and Ideas for Self-Compassion

Use these examples to inspire your daily intention-setting, affirmations, and self-compassion reminders. Feel free to choose from this list or create your own.

Daily Intention Settings

- Today, I will focus on being present.
- Today, I will practice patience with myself and others.
- Today, I will embrace change and adapt.
- Today, I will take moments to breathe deeply and reset.
- Today, I will be open to joy and gratitude.

Daily Affirmations

- I am worthy of care and healing.
- I trust my progress, even in small steps.
- I am resilient and can handle what comes my way.
- I deserve moments of peace and tranquility.
- I am enough, just as I am.

Self-Compassion Reminders

- I am doing my best, and that is enough.
- It's okay to have tough days; I will treat myself with kindness.
- I deserve love and understanding from myself.
- I allow myself to rest and recover without guilt.

Your Chance to Make a Difference

Healing is within your reach. Remember that it's an ongoing journey, and celebrate each small win as it happens. Every step forward is important, and each one brings you closer to breaking free from your trauma. Take a few moments now to help more people discover somatic therapy and feel the same benefits.

Simply by sharing your honest opinion of this book and a little about your own experience, you'll show new readers where they can find this information and begin their own healing journeys.

WANT TO HELP OTHERS?

Thank you so much for your support. You're making a real difference.

Scan the QR code below

CONCLUSION

Wow, what a journey we've taken in this book together! We've covered so much ground—from the first steps of understanding somatic therapy to exploring practical exercises and healing techniques. The heart of this book has always been aiming to simplify complex somatic therapy concepts and offer you practical steps to help manage trauma, PTSD, anxiety, and chronic pain.

I hope the tools and insights shared here are as transformative for you as they are for me.

Throughout this journey, we've kept a trauma-informed focus, minimizing the risk of re-traumatization. I have aimed to blend physical, mental, and emotional healing practices into a seamless, holistic approach to well-being. We also emphasized mindfulness techniques and self-compassion, knowing their importance in building emotional resilience, body awareness, and long-lasting healing.

Let's take a quick stroll down memory lane and revisit the major points we covered in each chapter:

In **Chapter 1**, we laid the foundations of somatic therapy. We explored its principles, history, and various modalities, understanding how this body-centered approach can lead to profound emotional and physical healing. The science behind the mind-body connection was also a key focus, with practical exercises like grounding and body awareness techniques.

Chapter 2 focused on emotional and physical healing techniques. We explored breathwork, yoga, Tai Chi, and Pilates, each offering unique benefits for managing stress and enhancing body awareness. This chapter provided step-by-step instructions and modifications to tailor these practices to your needs.

In **Chapter 3**, we crafted a customizable 28-day healing program. This chapter guided you through designing a personalized plan, incorporating daily 10-minute practices, and adapting techniques for different conditions like PTSD, anxiety, and chronic pain. Tracking progress and adjusting your plan were also vital aspects we discussed.

Chapter 4 focused on mindfulness techniques and emotional resilience. We learned about different types of mindfulness meditation, body scan exercises, and practical exercises for building resilience. This chapter emphasized the importance of staying present and managing emotions effectively.

Chapter 5 encompassed self-compassion and self-regulation. We explored the role of self-compassion in healing, practical exercises like journaling and reflection, and techniques for managing triggers and emotional states. Integrating self-compassion into daily life was a key takeaway from this chapter.

In **Chapter 6**, we explored real-time biofeedback and tech-based tools. We explored Heart Rate Variability Biofeedback (HRVB) and mindfulness apps, integrating these tools into your healing routine for enhanced self-awareness and emotional regulation.

Chapter 7 introduced advanced somatic practices, including advanced breathwork techniques, Somatic Experiencing (SE), and Polyvagal Theory. We also explored embodiment practices, emphasizing the importance of fully inhabiting your body for deeper healing.

Chapter 8 focused on integrating somatic practices into daily life. We discussed creating a somatic-friendly environment at home, establishing daily rituals, and balancing work, life, and somatic practices. This chapter emphasized the importance of making a supportive environment and engaging in consistent practices.

In **Chapter 9**, we highlighted the importance of community and support. We explored finding and joining support groups, building a support network with friends, family, and therapists, and engaging with online communities. The joy and growth in sharing stories of your journey and the power of collective healing were key themes.

Chapter 10 showcased transformational success stories and case studies. We learned from the experiences of individuals who have overcome PTSD, anxiety, and chronic pain through somatic therapy. These stories highlighted the power of resilience and the effectiveness of the techniques we discussed.

Finally, **Chapter 11** explored how to sustain the benefits of somatic therapy and highlighted the importance of consistent practices like mindfulness, movement, and self-reflection. It also provided practical tips for integrating self-care into daily life and overcoming challenges. We learned how to adjust healing plans, stay motivated, and engage with evolving somatic practices for ongoing growth and resilience.

A Continuing Journey

Healing is an ongoing and continuous path paved with small, consistent steps that cultivate a deeper connection with your mind and body. Like a garden tended with care, your healing will unfold in its own time, with moments of blossoming, growth, and renewal.

So, what's next? Begin by planting the seeds of the practices you have learned about here that resonated most with you. Track your progress, revisit your healing plan regularly, and surround yourself with supportive people and communities.

In closing, please know this *with all your being:*

You are capable of incredible transformation. The strength you need is already within you, and the tools in this book are here to guide and support you along the way. Each mindful breath and every act of self-compassion nurtures growth. Trust that, even in seasons of challenge, the seeds you've planted are quietly taking root beneath the surface.

Thank you for allowing me to be part of your life's journey. Here's to your life filled with healing, balance, and joy—one that reflects the love and beauty within you.

You've got this, and I'll be cheering you on every step of the way.

REFERENCES

Arlington Thrive. (n.d.). *Create a calming home environment for better mental health.* https://arlingtonthrive.org/create-a-calming-home-environment-for-better-mental-health/

BodyMind Centering. (n.d.). *Bonnie Bainbridge Cohen.* https://www.bodymindcentering.com/about/

Cohen, S. (2020, September 28). *How daily rituals and routines can change your life.* Stress Less Co. https://stresslessco.com/blog/2020/9/28/how-daily-rituals-and-routines-can-change-your-life

Ergos Institute, Inc.™. (n.d.). *Ray's story—Ergos Institute, inc™ - Somatic Experiencing.* https://www.somaticexperiencing.com/rays-story

Frame Fitness. (n.d.). *How the Pilates mind-body connection works for you.* https://www.framefitness.com/blog/news/how-the-pilates-mind-body-connection-works-for-you

Global SACAP. (n.d.). *Somatic Experiencing, Polyvagal Theory, and trauma.* https://global.sacap.edu.za/blog/applied-psychology/somatic-experiencing-polyvagal-theory-and-trauma/

Greater Good Science Center. (n.d.). *How to choose a type of mindfulness meditation.* https://greatergood.berkeley.edu/article/item/how_to_choose_a_type_of_mindfulness_meditation

Harvard Gazette. (2018, April 12). *When science meets mindfulness.* https://news.harvard.edu/gazette/story/2018/04/harvard-researchers-study-how-mindfulness-may-change-the-brain-in-depressed-patients/

Harvard Health Publishing. (n.d.). *Tai chi and chronic pain.* https://www.health.harvard.edu/alternative-and-integrative-health/tai-chi-and-chronic-pain

Healthline. (n.d.). *Body scan meditation: Benefits and how to do it.* https://www.healthline.com/health/body-scan-meditation

Higher Logic Vanilla. (n.d.). *How to keep your online community safe.* https://vanilla.higherlogic.com/blog/how-to-keep-your-online-community-safe/

Hopkins Medicine. (n.d.). *Somatic self-care | Office of Well-Being.* https://www.hopkinsmedicine.org/office-of-well-being/connection-support/somatic-self-care

Insight Timer. (n.d.). *Tai chi and Qigong for the treatment and prevention of ....* https://www.ncbi.nlm.nih.gov/pmc/articles/PMC3917559/

Khiron Clinics. (n.d.). *What is neuroplasticity, and how can it help in recovery?* https://khironclinics.com/blog/what-is-neuroplasticity-and-how-can-it-help-in-recovery/

Kripalu Center for Yoga & Health. (n.d.). *How yoga helps heal trauma: A Q&A with Bessel van der Kolk.* https://kripalu.org/resources/how-yoga-helps-heal-trauma-qa-bessel-van-der-kolk

Meridian Biofeedback. (n.d.). *Integrating mindfulness and biofeedback in the treatment ....*

https://meridian.allenpress.com/biofeedback/article/46/2/37/113475/Integrating-Mindfulness-and-Biofeedback-in-the

Mayo Clinic. (n.d.). *Support groups: Make connections, get help.* https://www.mayoclinic.org/healthy-lifestyle/stress-management/in-depth/support-groups/art-20044655

Mindfulness Exercises. (n.d.). *How mindfulness builds resilience: What science says.* https://mindfulnessexercises.com/how-mindfulness-builds-resilience-what-science-says/

MUIH. (n.d.). *Tending ourselves: Self-care strategies for sustainable work-life balance.* https://muih.edu/tending-ourselves-self-care-strategies-for-sustainable-work-life-balance/

National Center for Biotechnology Information (NCBI). (n.d.). *Brief structured respiration practices enhance mood and ....* https://www.ncbi.nlm.nih.gov/pmc/articles/PMC9873947/

National Center for Biotechnology Information (NCBI). (n.d.). *Heart rate variability biofeedback: How and why does it work?* https://www.ncbi.nlm.nih.gov/pmc/articles/PMC4104929/

National Center for Biotechnology Information (NCBI). (n.d.). *Mindfulness and emotion regulation: Insights from ....* https://www.ncbi.nlm.nih.gov/pmc/articles/PMC5337506/

National Center for Biotechnology Information (NCBI). (n.d.). *Somatic experiencing – Effectiveness and key factors of a ....* https://www.ncbi.nlm.nih.gov/pmc/articles/PMC8276649/

National Institutes of Health (NIH). (n.d.). *Emotional wellness toolkit.* https://www.nih.gov/health-information/emotional-wellness-toolkit

Porges, S. W. (n.d.). *Stephen W. Porges, PhD | Polyvagal Theory.* https://www.stephenporges.com/

Positive Psychology. (n.d.). *8 powerful self-compassion exercises & worksheets ....* https://positivepsychology.com/self-compassion-exercises-worksheets/

Positive Psychology. (n.d.). *Somatic experiencing therapy: 10 best exercises.* https://positivepsychology.com/somatic-experiencing/

Proactive Mental Wellness. (n.d.). *The role of trauma support groups in recovery.* https://proactivementalwellness.com/the-role-of-support-groups-in-trauma-recovery/

Psych Central. (n.d.). *Somatic therapy: How it works, uses, types, and ....* https://psychcentral.com/blog/how-somatic-therapy-can-help-patients-suffering-from-psychological-trauma

Recovery Center USA. (n.d.). *The importance of mental health check-ins: Raising awareness.* https://therecoverycenterusa.com/the-importance-of-mental-health-check-ins-raising-awareness/

SpiritVibez. (n.d.). *Breathwork to release trauma: 5 life-changing techniques.* https://spiritvibez.com/breathwork-to-release-trauma/

Stellar. (n.d.). *My movement: How Pilates transformed my self-confidence.* https://stellar.ie/real-talk/wellness/my-movement-how-pilates-transformed-my-self-confidence/119245

30 Best Peter Levine Quotes With Image. Bookey. Last modified September 12, 2023. https://www.bookey.app/quote-author/peter-levine

UCI Susan Samueli Integrative Health Institute. (n.d.). *7 strategies to make lifestyle changes that last.* https://ssihi.uci.edu/news-and-media/blog/7-strategies-to-make-lifestyle-changes-that-last/

Verywell Mind. (n.d.). *Grounding techniques for coping with PTSD and anxiety.* https://www.verywellmind.com/grounding-techniques-for-ptsd-2797300

White Horse Active. (n.d.). *A guide to mindful movement & its health benefits.* https://www.whitehorseactive.com/blogs/movementum-by-whitehorse/a-guide-to-mindful-movement-its-health-benefits?srsltid=AfmBOopNaxMRcyHQX-Or67e32fEVxZQejFvlJKecdKHMoGFmErcPiJdVa